Josie's Story

Josie's Story

Sorrel King

Atlantic Monthly Press
New York

Excerpt from "The Sound of Music" © 1965 Courtesy of Twentieth Century Fox. Written by Ernest Lehman. All rights reserved.

Excerpt from "Baby Beluga" © 1980 Homeland Publishing (SOCAN)/ Administered by Bug Music. All Rights Reserved. Used by Permission. Words and Music by Raffi Cavoukian and Debi Pike.

Published simultaneously in Canada
Printed in the United States of America

FIRST EDITION

ISBN-13: 978-0-8021-1920-9

Atlantic Monthly Press
an imprint of Grove/Atlantic, Inc.
841 Broadway
New York, NY 10003
Distributed by Publishers Group West
www.groveatlantic.com
09 10 11 12 13   10 9 8 7 6 5 4 3 2 1

To Tony, Jack, Relly, Eva, and Sam
and to all the doctors, nurses, and health-care providers
who go to work every day
to make lives better, and most of all
to Josie

Author's Note: In this book I have tried to the best of my memory to portray people, conversations, and events as they happened. Some names and places have been changed for reasons of privacy.

When it's dark enough, you can see the stars.

—Persian proverb

Josie's Story

The Picture

I took the lens cap off my new Nikon thirty-five millimeter camera that Tony had given me for my birthday and stood on the porch of the beach house, looking across the lawn to the ocean. The sun was beginning to lower itself toward the horizon, casting a warm glow onto Middle Pier, the dock we swam at every day. It was the last day of summer vacation. The bikes were on the back of the car, the refrigerator had been emptied, and the bags were ready to be loaded into the car the next morning before we caught a 7:00 a.m. ferry off the island.

"Look at the light," I said to Tony as I squinted through the camera lens. "It's perfect. Do you think we can get a Christmas card?"

He walked over and stood next to me. "You know how they hate it when you take their picture," he said. He looked at the four children swinging in the hammock. "We're gonna have to trick 'em." We handed them each a small plastic bag and told them we'd go on one last sea glass hunt.

Six-year-old Jack and five-year-old Relly grabbed the bags and raced down the dirt road to the pier. As I reached down to pick up Eva, who was three, her younger sister Josie pushed her away, grabbed my leg, and said, "mine, mine, mine." Josie had just turned one and, being the youngest of four, she had figured out early on how to get her way. Tony stooped down and threw Eva onto his shoulders just as she was about to give Josie a shove. He trotted behind Jack and Relly, Eva bouncing up and down on his shoulders. All three held their bags up to the sky, filling them with air. I followed behind with the camera slung around my neck and Josie in my arms.

When we got to the beach we told them that we'd look for sea glass later. "You guys sit on the bench and let me take a few pictures."

They knew they had been tricked and immediately started complaining.

"Don't you want to have a nice picture for Santa Claus?" I asked. They followed me to the end of the dock and sat on the white bench with sour looks on their faces.

The "say cheese" thing never seemed to work when it came to picture taking; neither did "cheeseburger." Even switching to more enticing words like "I love Christmas" or "Santa Claus" never seemed to tickle them enough to force their lips into smiles for the camera. We needed real comedy to make the four King children stop poking each other, stop whining, and smile.

"Are you ready?" Tony asked as I pulled out the camera.

"Yep," I said, stepping back five paces. Tony danced and made silly faces behind me as I looked through the camera lens waiting to catch a smile.

"Are you getting any good ones?" he asked. I could hear him jumping around.

"No, they're not laughing."

"I know what'll work."

The children and I watched him run down the dock. He grabbed something from the beach and ran back, hiding it behind him.

"Okay, get ready," he said.

I held the camera up to my eye, finger poised, and watched through the lens as the four children began to laugh. I could feel drops of water on my neck as Tony dangled wet seaweed over my head, then lay bits of it on my shoulders, and I yelled at him helplessly to stop. I was getting smiles, but waiting for the wind to stop blowing Relly's hair in her face, waiting for Eva to take her finger out of her mouth.

I lowered the camera and paused to watch Josie grab her brother's shoulder and stand up. She spread her chubby legs, balancing herself perfectly, and looked at me. There it was. Four children smiling and laughing, the soft summer sun setting on their happy faces. I pushed the auto-focus button and snapped, capturing the perfect moment. That was the last picture I took of my four children together.

Six months later, Josie was dead and our lives as we had known them were over. The photograph would be pasted onto the little wooden box that held Josie's ashes and would be buried far beneath the ground. The same photo would be flashed on screens behind me as I spoke to hundreds and thousands of health care providers from all over the world. For the months and years following Josie's death, it hurt to look at the picture, to see Josie's face. It hurt to think about that day on Middle Pier.

It was not a typical family portrait with hair ribbons, pretty dresses, slicked-back hair, and blazers. It was *our* family portrait. Relly is shrieking in laughter and pushing her tangled hair out of her face as her father, who is also laughing, plops more seaweed onto my head. Jack is turning his head to look at her. Eva is scrunching her knees up under her light-blue sundress and has taken her finger out of her mouth.

And Josie is standing firm in her plastic lion sandals, one arm against her side as if at any minute she might raise it and say, "Okay, pick me up now." In her other hand she is clutching a soggy graham cracker that has oozed all over her pale green sundress. Her brown hair is held back by a yellow clip that Relly put in moments before. She is gazing steadily at the camera, through the lens and into my eyes. She is cocking her head and smiling at me, a half smile.

It's been six years since she died. When I look at the picture now, I no longer feel searing pain. I can marvel at how Jack, Relly, and Eva have grown. Still, Josie's eyes seem to look through me. Holding the picture close and looking into her serene, smiling face, I can't help but wonder if that day on the pier she knew something the rest of us didn't.

1

I was draining the spaghetti at our home in Richmond, Virginia, Josie sat in her swing playing with her little blue bear.

The phone rang and I could hear the excitement in Tony's voice when I picked up. A few weeks earlier he had been asked to run his bank's sales trading desk. It was a great opportunity for a thirty-two-year-old, but meant moving to Baltimore, where the company was headquartered. He was there now, in search of the perfect home. He had called to tell me he had found it.

"The house is old and definitely needs some work, but the land around it is beautiful," he said.

"So, is it a total dump or what?" I asked, pouring the spaghetti sauce onto the noodles.

"Well, yeah sort of," he admitted. He told me it had been a barn in the 1800s and then, in 1920, it had been converted into a house. "It's got green shingles and huge windows with that old, wavy glass that you like. If we want it, we need to sign the contract today."

"But what about the inside?" I asked.

"We can check it out during the inspection. If we wait until then, we'll lose it. It's the land. There's something about it that's kind of magical. It reminds me of Bruce Farm."

"Bruce Farm? It reminds you of Bruce Farm?"

"Yeah, it does. It really does," he said. "You're going to fall in love with this place."

In 1939, my mother's parents, in search of a summer escape from the city life of Washington, DC, found it when they stepped foot onto an old farm that sat at the top of the Blue Ridge Mountains in Loudoun County, Virginia. The huge stone house with flagstone terraces, called the Big House, was surrounded by sprawling open lawns of Kentucky bluegrass. Fieldstone walls separated the manicured lawns from the pastures that were grazed by Black Angus cattle and horses. But the thing that took my grandparents' breath away when they stood on the farm for the first time was the view. From the front porch, I came to see and love what they saw that day: a pale green lawn gently sloping down to a stone wall, above which a panoramic view of multiple shades of blue burst as far as the eye could see, making you feel as if you were looking over the ocean. With a slight squint, you could see dairy farms, little towns, and country roads. With a telescope you could see the Washington Monument in the solid, earthy valley. This was God's country, and its name was Bruce Farm.

Bruce Farm was where my mother and her sister spent their summers and weekends, and as children my siblings and I did, too. It was a place where we were taught, like my mother had been, the meaning of hard work. Our mornings were spent weeding the vegetable garden, mucking out stalls, creosoting fences, and blazing trails. When the work was done we'd pull on our bathing suits, lace up our work boots, and run as fast as we could, with towels flying like superhero capes, across the lawn, over the stone wall, and down the dirt road to jump into the cool pond. Bruce Farm held a special place in all of our hearts.

Tony had been to Bruce Farm, and it got to him the same way it got to me. So, I could tell, as he described what he saw walking around the property in Baltimore, that he had fallen for the place for the same reasons that he knew I would, and that no matter how dilapidated the house was it would become our new home.

"Josie, it looks like we're going to live in an old green barn. What do you think about that?" I said, plopping a zwieback biscuit on the tray of her swing. She liked the Swiss cardboard-like crackers and sucked on them until they became mushy enough to squeeze in her fists. When she wanted a fresh one, she'd throw the wad of mush at Trapper, the smelly, thirteen-year-old Lab that no one in the family paid attention to anymore except Josie, who adored him. He'd catch the mush that came flying his way and she'd laugh from her swing, kick out her feet, and dangle her chubby zwieback-encrusted fingers in front of him. He'd lick them clean.

Josie was the youngest of four, our caboose. When I was a little girl, I always wanted to have four children. Maybe because I was one of four it was the perfect, even number, not too big, not too small. I loved being part of a big family. Everyone always had someone to play with; no one was ever left out. A life like *The Brady Bunch* or *Eight Is Enough* was right up my alley: the more confusion, the more chaos, the better.

With the birth of each of our children, driving home from the hospital was like Christmas morning. Everything was magical. But with Josie, there was more. It was July 3, a typical sweltering, humid, Virginia summer day. My mother insisted on driving, so the three of us—Tony, two-day-old Josie, and I—sat in the back seat as she slowly—ten miles below the speed limit, holding her breath, gritting her teeth, gripping the steering wheel—made her way down the highway.

I looked at Josie's tiny cheeks as she lay swaddled in the pink blanket that the hospital had given us. She had brown eyes and lots of brown hair with a cowlick that threw part of her hair straight up. Somehow, we had wedged her into the car seat without waking her. I was making mental notes, thinking that I had better tuck this away in the memory bank because this was it. No more babies. Josie completed us. I looked at Tony, who was smiling as he gazed down at Josie, probably having the same thought. Jack, Relly, and Eva were at home waiting for their new little sister. Soon we would all be together, at home for the first time. Four children. Perfect.

Richmond was home for me, where I had grown up and where my parents still lived, along with my brother, Mac, and sister Mary Earle. My younger sister Margaret was right up the road in Washington, DC. Tony and I had spent the previous year building a house in the country just outside of town, on a pretty slice of land next to my parents. From our house the children could walk down a little hill and then up a little hill and be at their grandparents, Big Rel and Pop's doorstep.

We had loved our home with its dark gray shingles and front porch that faced the western sky; nothing but horse pastures and hay fields framed our view as the sun set every evening. I had planted a bed of perennials and a tiny Carolina jasmine vine with hopes that the vine would climb up the front pillar of the house and shade the porch with fragrant yellow flowers. We had lived there for a little over a year when Tony was offered the promotion in Baltimore.

Our life in the countryside of Virginia was perfect, but Tony and I both agreed that we were too young to say to ourselves: *this is where we'll be forever.* The children were not yet entrenched in school and so we decided to take a chance. It would be an adventure, we told ourselves. "We can rent the house in Virginia out and if we don't like Baltimore we can come home," Tony promised me. And so we decided to leave our family and friends and the home that we had worked so hard to build, and start a new life in Baltimore.

A few weeks after Tony had signed the contract, we drove to Baltimore to look at our new house—a house I had never seen. My parents took care of Jack, Relly, and Eva, and we took Josie so that I could continue nursing her. Tony and I had been to Baltimore together once before and had spent no more than a few hours with the realtor, driving around the neighborhoods, trying to get a feel for the place. Here we were, buying a house, knowing practically nothing about the city.

It was early October when we turned onto Kayhill Lane, in Baltimore. Through the changing leaves I saw a rolling lawn topped by a pretty, green-shingled farmhouse, shaped like a saltbox, with a gambrel roof and an awkward hay-bale-pitching window in the center.

In the mailbox we found a note from the current owner.

Dear Tony and Sorrel,
  I hope this old house provides you with many happy memories. In the early 1900s, it was a barn and was called Ashline.
  Sincerely,
Elizabeth Cunningham

A house with a name. This was going to be good. I strapped Josie into her front carrier and we headed in with the realtor.

It was inspection day and lots of people scurried about carrying clipboards. The living room was amazing: high ceilings, an old mantelpiece, and a bay window flanked by huge windows, each with twelve panes of beautiful, old, wavy glass, just like Tony had said. It helped that Mrs. Cunningham, who hadn't moved out yet, had good taste, and this room was a showcase of her antiques and artwork. The dining room was equally as elegant, with two large French doors that opened out onto a redbrick terrace. This was definitely a grown-up house, and I was not quite sure what we were doing in it. I was beginning to wonder why no one else had bought the place.

The realtor saved the worst for last—the worst being the rest of the house. The kitchen was tiny, split into three little sections. There was no place for a kitchen table and hardly any room to cook. Most appalling of all, there was green carpet everywhere. As we moved upstairs the situation did not improve. The bathrooms had various wires sticking out, the bedrooms were small, and the hallways were slanted, giving the doorways a cockeyed look. The basement had signs of water damage. Ashline was not looking so hot anymore.

"Do you think there's any way we can get out of this?" I whispered into Tony's ear.

"It's not so bad. We can live with it and then fix it up," he said as Josie reached for him. He took her from me and led me outside. "You're going to love this part."

Hearing Tony, the realtor took his cue. "Don't you love it?" he asked a little too enthusiastically, leaning close to me with bright, excited eyes. "I've got the name of a great contractor who can fix some of this stuff," he added, holding the front door open for me.

The land *was* spectacular and as I walked around looking at the old boxwoods, the pretty dogwoods, the tulip poplars, the ash tree that longed to have swings hanging from its branches, and the rolling lawns I could see why Tony had fallen for the place. Along with the house came a little barn that backed on to Lake Roland, an old city reservoir that had lots of walking paths around it. The view out of every window made you feel as if you were in the country, yet the schools were five minutes away and there was a Starbucks practically within walking distance.

"Should we go for it?" Tony asked, handing Josie back to me.

As we stood on the redbrick terrace looking over the lawn, I could feel a hint of Bruce Farm about the old place. I told him I was in if he was.

"What do you think of your new house, little monkey?" Tony said, squeezing Josie's yellow-socked feet as he leaned down to give her a kiss on the cheek. He put his arm around me and we stood there, the three of us. "I think we're gonna like it here," he said.

As we headed to the car the inspectors informed us that we better take a good look at the Terminix contract because there was definitely some termite damage in the front portion of the house.

"Don't worry," the realtor said. "My contractor does termites, too."

2

We settled into our new life in Baltimore. Jack, Relly, and Eva were happy at their new school, Tony was enjoying his job, and I stayed busy at home with Josie, trying to fix up the old house. Although I was liking Baltimore, I missed Richmond terribly. It was a happy surprise when, one day in late January of 2001, we pulled into the driveway to find a green Explorer with Virginia plates parked in front of the farmhouse. "Hey guys, what's that license plate say?" I asked.

Five-year-old Relly leaned up front to get a closer look. "Bbb-iiii-gggg," she said, sounding out each letter as her kindergarten teachers had taught her. "Rrrr . . . eeeee . . ."

Jack, her brother, who was a year older, quickly unrolled his window and craned his neck to get a closer look. He was not about to let her beat him to it.

"Jack, let Relly figure it out. She's almost got it," I said, as I pulled the dark blue Suburban up next to the Explorer.

"Big Rel! It says Big Rel. That's Big Rel's car. Big Rel is here!" he blurted out.

"Big Rel, that's right!" Relly added excitedly as she struggled to climb out of the car. She and Jack raced to the house as three-year-old Eva trailed behind, trying her best to keep her blue fleece blanket up off the ground with one hand while sucking a finger on her other. I unbuckled seventeen-month-old Josie from her car seat and followed them into the house, carrying all of the backpacks, coats, and snack wrappers that they had left behind. My mother—or Big Rel as the children had nicknamed her—had surprised us with a visit.

My mother was, and still is, a beautiful woman. In her younger years people said she looked like Jackie O. Some said she was prettier. "I know I should have called," she said, bending over to hug the children, then standing up to take Josie from me, "but Pop was out of town so I thought I'd drive up and see what you guys were up to." The children sat on the sofa with their grandmother and began telling her about their new school, their new bedrooms, and how I had let them paint the old kitchen cabinets before the workmen took them out and put them in the Dumpster.

"We don't have a kitchen anymore," Jack said.

"We get to go out to dinner all the time," Relly added as Eva, still sucking her finger and holding her blanket, wedged herself onto Big Rel's lap next to Josie, who tried unsuccessfully to push her away.

She hadn't been to see us since we had started renovations on the old green-shingled farmhouse, which was still a work in progress. I gave her a tour, pointing out where new walls would be going, where doors and windows would be placed, and where the new kitchen would be. She carried Josie, stepping over two-by-fours and piles of plywood with Jack, Relly, and Eva following behind.

"This looks like more work than building a house from scratch," she said. "How on earth are you going to live like this?"

"Let's just finish the tour," I said, leading her through the framing of the family room, mudroom, and bathroom.

We showed her the old, still-intact dining room, which was now serving as kitchen, family room, dining room, and play room.

"Isn't this nice and cozy," I asked as I began laying kindling and logs in the fireplace. "It's like living in a cabin." I struck a match and lit the fire.

"How long will this take?" she asked.

"I don't know, six months or so."

She looked suspiciously at the makeshift stove and the milk crates filled with flour, sugar, and cereal boxes. I recognized this look, her head cocked, brows furrowed, and mouth twisted; it was the same one she had used when I was a teenager and wore feather earrings and ripped jeans.

The children sat down to color and start their homework as Josie pushed the "ON" button to her little music cube and began her knee-buckle dance. She had gotten the toy for Christmas and loved dancing to the *"I love you, you love me"* Barney song. After ten minutes of it being played over and over it began to drive us all crazy. We had searched for the volume control but there was none.

Jack marched over, grabbed the toy from Josie, and turned it off. Josie shrieked, grabbed a handful of his hair, and burst into tears. Screaming, Jack tried to dislodge himself, but Josie pulled harder. I pried back her little fingers and released Jack from her iron grip. She cried until I picked her up and let her push the button back on.

"You're spoiling her. You should put her in time-out," Jack said.

"You're right, but she's so little, and look how cute she is. You used to do the same thing when you were her age, and you turned out okay."

Big Rel announced she was going to take a bubble bath and that whoever showed her where there was a tub that actually worked would get to pour the bubbles in. They all raced upstairs, leaving me alone with the Barney song pulsing in my ears.

The children loved sitting on the floor and talking to Big Rel as she lay back in the bath in her skirted bathing suit, covered up to her neck in bubbles. Eva and Relly brought in their Barbies—the ones that had not yet had all their hair cut off—for shampooing. Big Rel let them pour more bubbles in and told funny stories. This time it was even more of a treat because she was using a bathroom that had never been used before. It was across the hall from Josie's room and had been closed for renovations. There wasn't much in it that worked other than the old tub. Josie brought in all of her bath toys including her favorite, a little blue airplane.

At about six, Tony arrived with take-out Thai food and was opening up a bottle of wine when my mother reappeared with the children all in their pajamas. "Big Rel, it's good to see you," he said, handing her a glass of wine. "What do you think of the house?"

"I think you all have your work cut out for you," she said, taking a sip of the wine as they stood together in front of the fireplace.

"I know, but when it's all done it'll be great," he said. "Next year we'll have a big Thanksgiving with you and Pop and all the cousins."

Josie wiggled off my lap and walked over to her music

square. Jack and Relly were fed up with the song, and as it started to play they went upstairs to our bedroom to watch a cartoon.

My mother adored Tony and when the two were together I was often a fly on the wall. I listened to their conversation, sometimes interjecting, as I dished the Thai food onto paper plates.

"Where'd Josie go?" asked Tony.

We hadn't noticed that the music had stopped.

"I think she went upstairs to watch TV," I replied.

I was walking up the steps to check when I heard Josie let out a piercing scream. I started running. My legs couldn't carry me fast enough. She was standing next to the bathtub, screaming, with her eyes squeezed shut and arms jutting out from her sides. She was soaking wet. I ripped off the pajamas. Her skin was bright red and starting to blister. I grabbed a towel, wrapped her in it, and looked in the tub. I saw the water, and the airplane. I stuck my hand in. It was hot, scalding hot. I screamed for Tony to call 911.

I tried to piece together what had just occurred. Josie must have followed her siblings upstairs and, instead of joining them to watch *Rugrats,* she had taken a detour to the bathroom to find her blue airplane. She had probably wanted to see it float again, so she turned the knob closest to her little arm. The one with the "H" on it. Then she must have climbed in with her airplane. I felt my throat tighten. I had taken my eyes off her.

The ambulance arrived and the paramedics took Josie from me, laid her down, and unwrapped her. The skin on her legs and arms was red and oozy. She lay crying as the paramedics wrapped her in gauze. They put her in the ambulance and I jumped in, too, screaming for Tony to get me a bottle of milk. It was her bedtime, and she always had a bottle before going to sleep. He shoved the bottle in my bag and handed it all to me. "I'll follow you down there," he said. The ambulance doors slammed shut.

As the ambulance backed out of the driveway I could see the children and my mother through the window. They were sitting on the floor by the fireplace and she was handing Jack a board game. They were scared and confused, and their grandmother was trying to comfort and distract them.

"Everything is going to be just fine," she was probably saying. "Josie's going to a hospital and some nice doctors are going to fix her, and she'll be home soon. Let's play Chutes and Ladders, and I'll make some hot chocolate. Eva, you can go first since you're the youngest."

They must have been relieved. Of course Josie was going to be fine. Big Rel said so. It was as if time had stopped in that room, as if nothing else existed beyond the windows in the cold dark.

3

When we arrived at Johns Hopkins Bayview Medical Center we were met by two police officers, who walked alongside me as we headed toward the emergency room. They began asking me questions, but as I stopped to answer them I watched Josie and the paramedics disappear around a corner. I ran down the hall, chasing them, yelling to the police officers that I had to be with my daughter.

I knew very little about hospitals but one thing I did know was that Johns Hopkins was the best. I had never been in an emergency room before. It was a narrow room divided into sections by curtains. While we waited for the ER doctor, a nurse gave Josie a lollipop with pain medication. She quietly sucked on it while I stroked her head. I could hear the doctors, nurses, and paramedics in the surrounding bays taking care of other patients, one with a gunshot wound, one with severe chest pains, and another who had been in an automobile accident. The medical staff spoke quickly, the tension in their voices seeming to rise and fall each time a paramedic brought in a new patient. Controlled chaos surrounded me as Josie and I waited our turn.

The doctor was unable to get an IV into Josie's tiny veins and decided that Josie should be seen at the Johns Hopkins Children's Center. When we arrived, we were taken to the

PICU, pediatric intensive care unit on the seventh floor. While we waited for the doctor, I whispered "My Favorite Things," the *Sound of Music* song that I always sang to her at bedtime.

The doors blasted open and instead of seeing white coats with stethoscopes, I found myself face-to-face with the same two police officers who had followed me at Bayview.

"Mrs. King, can you please tell me what happened?" one asked. "What time, approximately, did your husband come home? And where were you and your husband when Josie turned on the water? Mrs. King, why was your mother in town?"

I answered their questions as they looked at me and took notes. I wondered why they were asking me these things.

The police officers left as the doctor came in. She told me to sit in the waiting room while they looked at Josie. I sat alone on the turquoise vinyl bench and stared at the blaring lights of the vending machine. It was 11:00 p.m. when Tony ran in.

"How is she?"

"She's okay," I said. "They're looking at her now. Where have you been? What took so long?"

"I had to talk to the police and show a detective around the house."

"That's weird. There were two policemen here asking me questions, too."

I was too confused and too worried about Josie to comprehend that a child abuse investigation was going on. The doctor came out and told us they were still trying to get the IV in. It was now 12:15 a.m.

An hour later we were told we could go be with her. She was wrapped in gauze and her eyes were closed. The doctor explained to us that she had first- and second-degree burns covering 60 percent of her body. They said that they would need to watch for infection, keep her well hydrated, and that she may need a skin graft or two but that she was stable. She would be okay.

I often think back to that night. I consider every detail, trying to figure out how things could have gone differently. If we hadn't given Josie the music box, she wouldn't have been listening to that song that night. Jack and Relly wouldn't have gone upstairs, and Josie wouldn't have followed them. Most of all I wonder how I allowed myself to let her out of my sight.

How could I have let this happen?

I sat in the hospital room staring at Josie wrapped in gauze, hooked up to an IV in a drug-induced sleep. All I could think of was that it should have been me. It should be me in the hospital bed with burns all over my body, not Josie. When I had my first child a great burden was lifted from my shoulders. I was no longer worried about dying. Instead, I had a new emotion to contend with: a crazy love more powerful than any love I had ever felt for anyone. I watched her eyelids flutter as she dreamed. I would have given anything to trade places with her.

Tony and I stayed by Josie's bed all night. I watched the sun rise and chase the darkness from the room, feeling the optimism that one feels whenever a new day begins. Josie was stable. She was getting fluids and nourishment. I wanted to get to work doing whatever I could so that Josie could come back home.

Tony went downstairs to the cafeteria to get us some coffee.

Soon after he had left, the doctor and the residents came into Josie's room and began discussing her care as I sat quietly.

"The first thing we need to do is think about *why* Josie is in here," the doctor said to the group.

She gave me an icy stare and the others in the room turned to look at me. It slowly began to dawn on me that these people thought Josie had been a victim of child abuse, abused by her parents. By me. My hope that the doctors and I would be a team, working together to heal my daughter, dissolved in this harsh realization. I stood by her bed, too afraid to move or speak for fear that this doctor would not give Josie the care she needed because she thought I had abused her.

Tony arrived just after they left. "What did the doctor say?" he asked, handing me a cup of coffee.

"They think we did this to her," I said. I ran the back of my fingers along Josie's soft cheek, letting the tears slide down my face. Tony was sitting on the other side of the bed. He stood up and walked over to me.

"Don't cry," he said. "It's going to be okay." He explained to me in a calm voice that when a child comes to the ER they have to ask these questions. "It's protocol," he said.

A young woman came in and introduced herself as Monica, the patient-service coordinator. She was a fast talker and explained that in an hour there was going to be a child protection service meeting, and we needed to be there. She would be back to escort us to the meeting. We nodded as she left the room and I looked at Tony. He read the panic in my eyes.

"They're just doing their job."

I was glad when Monica had left the room and we could be alone with Josie.

The nurse on duty was named Amy. She had long, pretty blonde hair that was pulled back into a ponytail that hung below her shoulder blades. She was the only one who treated me like what I was: a terrified mother who desperately loved her child.

I sat next to Josie and looked at the little electrodes stuck to her chest. I followed the lines up to the monitor that hung above her bed, trying to decipher what exactly it did. "It's called an electrocardiograph," Amy told me, as she walked over to Josie's bed. "An EKG. It monitors her heart rhythm, heart rate, and respiratory rate," she explained. I nodded my head.

I asked her what the clip on Josie's finger was for. "That's a Pulsox monitor," she said. "It registers the level of oxygen saturation." She explained to me that patients with burns often become hypermetabolic, which means their heart has to work extremely hard to pump blood and get oxygen, which is crucial in nourishing the body. When not enough oxygen is delivered, the body takes longer to heal. An alarm goes off when the pulse oximeter monitor detects a low oxygen saturation, signaling the nurse to give the patient supplemental oxygen, which is done by simply putting an oxygen mask up to the patient's airway.

And so Amy allowed me to be Pulsox monitor watcher. Every time the number got to a certain level I held the oxygen mask up to Josie's face before the alarm sounded.

I was grateful for my new job. It made me feel as if I was part of the team, as if I was contributing to her recovery. I saw how hard the nurses worked and how busy they always were. I felt honored to be helping them.

When I wasn't watching the monitors or holding an oxygen mask up to Josie's face I would lay my head next to hers and whisper songs in her ear. I stroked her forehead, hoping she could hear and feel me in her drug-clouded world.

Monica, the patient-service coordinator, returned with her clipboard and took us to the meeting. Not only was she a fast talker, she was a fast walker. We tried to keep up, dodging carts and people as she led us down the hall. She opened a door and ushered us into a small room that was mostly occupied by a large table and several chairs. She introduced us to the various members of the group and pointed to where we should sit. They stared at us as we took our seats. I looked down at what I was wearing—tan corduroys, a dark green sweater, and tennis shoes—the same clothes I had put on the morning before, when life was simple and my greatest concerns were getting the children to and from school and deciding what to make for dinner. I wondered if I looked like a mother who would abuse her child. Would Josie be taken away from us? Were the social service people at our house waiting for my mother to pack Jack's, Relly's, and Eva's bags and take them to a foster home? I came out of my haze to hear them thanking us for cooperating. The investigation had been completed; it was apparent to them that this was clearly a household accident.

I don't remember feeling any sort of huge relief for being cleared of the suspicion of child abuse, but I do remember feeling relieved that the meeting was over and that I could get back to Josie. Monica escorted us back to our room. She didn't walk so fast this time and seemed friendlier, asking us how Josie was doing and how old her siblings were.

It was 12:30 in the afternoon when we returned to Josie's room, and as day number two wore on the doctors and nurses who filtered through seemed to have changed their opinion of me. Their chilly demeanors had warmed and my spirits lifted. We were feeling optimistic enough that Tony went home to check on the other children and to bring back Josie's little blue bear and a tape recorder so that we could play her favorite songs.

By day number three, our new life in the Hopkins PICU was beginning to run like a well-oiled machine. Tony went back to work, coming to the hospital every day for a few hours after the stock market closed. My mother took care of Jack, Relly, and Eva, driving them to and from school while I stood watch over Josie.

I no longer kept track of the days of the week, the Mondays, Tuesdays and Wednesdays. My calendar was now a counting of the days spent at the hospital: day one, day two, day three. By day four, I had built a routine around the doctors' and nurses' shifts. At seven o'clock every morning, there would be a shift change, during which the nurse who was about to leave would update the new nurse, debriefing her on each body system including cardiac, respiratory, and digestive. Usually parents were not allowed to sit in on these debriefings, but as time went on, and as the nurses got to know me, I was included.

I would stand and listen as they discussed Josie. "Her oxygen saturation has increased, at 0500 we switched to a nasal cannula," the nurse said, turning to me to explain, "that means her breathing is almost normal and there is no need for a breathing mask." I nodded my head. "Her blood cultures are all no-growth to date." She looked at me again and explained that this meant Josie was clear of infections. I was grateful to the nurses for letting me be a part of their team and for taking the extra time to explain things to me.

Most mornings I would walk down the long corridor in the basement to buy a cup of coffee and a muffin for myself and the nurse on duty. On the walls were large, framed posters, one after the other, gallery-like, of the consecutive covers of the *U.S. News & World Report* proclaiming Johns Hopkins the best hospital in the country. It was like being in a museum and looking at the most amazing artwork you have ever seen and having the artist right there in the room with you. These doctors and nurses who raced by me every morning were some of the best in their fields. I was in awe of them and their work. Josie was in a good place.

Baltimore is known for two things: Maryland crabs and the Johns Hopkins Hospital. Actually three things, if you throw in lacrosse. Watching the workings of the hospital from within, witnessing the doctors and nurses at work, I understood why Baltimoreans are proud of the place.

The hospital sits in the heart of East Baltimore, a stone's throw from the downtown financial district and minutes from the city's inner harbor. Its sidewalks buzz with a combination of white coats, blue scrubs, dark suits, and homeless people trying to make a few bucks. Orange and yellow detour signs continually change the traffic pattern around Hopkins, while construction vehicles add to the overall congestion.

The Hopkins medical campus is a sprawling maze of buildings that are home to extraordinary teaching and healing.

Its famous dome sits atop one of the original hospital buildings on an old cobblestone street. It was in this place, in 1889,
that the hospital was opened, thanks to a charitable bequest
by a wealthy businessman named Johns Hopkins.

A few years later in 1893, the Johns Hopkins University
School of Medicine opened. These Hopkins medical institutions quickly became known for their pioneering medical
advancements. CPR and the use of rubber gloves during operations are among the many, many innovations begun at
Hopkins. It was the first teaching hospital in the country to
establish the modern concept of a residency program that for-
mally integrated teaching, research, and supervision by the
school of medicine faculty into the daily operations of the
hospital. So much of what modern medicine is today stems
from the old domed building overlooking East Baltimore.

Academic medical centers like Hopkins, as well as Yale,
Duke, the Cleveland Clinic, and the Mayo Clinic, operate as
systems in which care is delivered in what many in the health
care industry refer to as silo-like in form; that is, individual
specialty teams function separately from one another. There
may be a surgical team, a pain management team, a respiratory team, each made up of the best in their field. Although
these specialty teams are highly effective, the mere fact that
they operate somewhat independently can often lead to a
breakdown in the flow of communication.

A hierarchy, or pecking order of sorts, defines each of
these silos. Each department is captained by a chief, who
oversees that department's full-time specialists, known as
attending physicians. The attending physicians lead the
hands-on training of the fellows, the residents, and, at times,
the medical students. From the patient's perspective, it is

the attending physician who is the main point person, who oversees all of the care and who is ultimately responsible for treatment.

Beneath the attending is the fellow, who has completed his or her residency and is being further trained in a subspecialty, such as pediatrics, emergency medicine, or cardiology.

Beneath them are the residents, who commit to three to four years of post-medical-school training where the real hands-on learning lies. The years of residency are usually the toughest, with excruciating hours and intense information overload. This is the period during which those who are not 100 percent committed often quit.

Nurses inhabit the base of the pyramid. They are at the bedside 24/7 and tend to the everyday care of the patients. They must tolerate long hours and are often short-staffed. They see it all.

With systems like this, in which information flows vertically and horizontally and hundreds of exchanges occur every day between the doctors and nurses and their various teams, the chance for there to be a breakdown in the system is extremely high.

Somewhere in the midst of this complex system are the patient and the family, who try to make sense of it all, hoping that they will be heard along the way.

I had often wondered why one would choose to be treated at an academic hospital, where the patient is examined, poked, prodded, and diagnosed by students, doctors in training. What I learned as I spent my days at Hopkins was that academic hospitals offer the cutting edge in technology and therefore provide the resources for the discovery of the next gene, the cure for cancer, and the next miracle in which a life will be saved. These academic hospitals probe deeply into the world of healing and every step of the way articles are written in well-known medical journals where break-through information is shared so that other physicians can learn from it. A hospital such as Hopkins selects only the best: top attending surgeons such as Dr. Charles Paidas, and top fellows such as Dr. Amal Murarka and Dr. Milissa McKee. These talented doctors made up Josie's team and we became fast friends.

Like all surgeons, Dr. Paidas possessed several key traits: brilliance, the ability to make major split-second decisions, razor-sharp vision, and the steadiest of hands. If one were to stereotype a surgeon one might say that what amazing talents they possess in the operating room, they lack at the bedside. But Dr. Paidas was different. We liked him from the beginning. The first day that Tony and I met him, he gave us a piece of paper with his cell phone number, his pager number, and, scribbled at the bottom, his home phone number. "Call me anytime, day or night. Whatever you need or whatever questions you have, just call." He told us to call him Chuck.

He was personable, with a great sense of humor, and tall and olive skinned, with warm brown eyes, a mustache, and black hair sprinkled with some gray.

After Tony went back to work, my sister Margaret would often drive up from Washington to spend the day with Josie and me, and she took to Chuck, too.

"That's it, that's who he reminds me of, the surgeon in *Corelli's Mandolin*," Margaret said one morning as we sat on either side of Josie, massaging her hands with Bacitracin, an ointment that keeps the skin from getting dry and guards against infections. She told me the book was about a handsome, charismatic surgeon who lived in a small village on a Greek island during World War II. People traveled far and wide to be cured by him. While she was talking Chuck walked into the room.

"How's she doing?" he asked as he washed his hands.

I gave him an update, telling him her urine output and potassium level. Margaret told him that the monitor on her finger kept slipping off.

Chuck smiled at us. "It looks like you two might have a career in health care after all of this."

He put on his rubber gloves and began unwrapping Josie's wounds. I liked the way he touched her, gentle and precise, always looking at her face for any signs of discomfort. As he examined her he explained to me exactly what he was doing and why.

"These wounds are healing nicely," he said as his pager began beeping. He continued to work on Josie while it beeped until finally he raised his gloved hands and asked me to reach into his pocket and grab the pager.

I looked at Chuck's pockets and then at Margaret on the other side of the bed and wondered which pocket the beeping was coming from.

"Right here," he said, pointing with his elbow.

I reached into the pocket of his white coat and quickly grabbed the beeper, relieved that it was not in his pants pocket. He asked me to read him the message and I did, feeling honored to be helping this brilliant doctor, and as he continued to examine Josie I stood beside him trying to learn from his every move.

Margaret asked him if he had read *Corelli's Mandolin*.

He had heard of it, but not yet read it. She told him about the book and the Greek surgeon.

"He reminds me of you," she said to him.

"He cures everyone," I added. "Just like you."

Dr. McKee, the surgical fellow, was Chuck's right hand, his protégée. Not only was she brilliant, she was beautiful and tall, with long blonde hair and skin like porcelain. Everyone moved aside when she walked down the hall, especially the young residents. She commanded respect and, from what the nurses told me, she deserved every ounce of it.

She had graduated from college when she was just fifteen, receiving a BA from the University of Minnesota. She went on to pursue her dream of becoming a doctor and received her medical degree from the University of North Dakota when she was only nineteen. She was a genius, a child prodigy. During the next ten years she would receive her master's of public health from Johns Hopkins University, complete her surgical residency at Loma Linda University Medical Center, and become a pediatric surgery fellow at Johns Hopkins.

I watched her closely as she spoke to the residents, most of whom looked to be a good bit older than she. They followed her around with their clipboards, jotting down the bits of brilliance that she threw their way.

When she came into Josie's room she was efficient and professional, flipping through charts, scanning computer screens, looking closely at Josie and always asking me if I had any questions or concerns. Milissa was not overly sociable and even seemed a bit shy, but she was kind and when I got to know her I found she was actually quite funny. Sometimes Margaret and I would engage her with questions about her beautiful skin and whether she had a boyfriend or not. She opened up to us and at times we would all talk like old friends.

But it was Dr. Murarka, the pediatric fellow, with whom I felt closest. Late in the afternoon of day two after I'd already met him a few times, I stepped out of Josie's room for a few minutes while Tony watched over her. I was standing with my back to the elevators, looking out the window so that no one could see me as I silently cried. I could hear people waiting for the elevator, talking, behind me.

"Are you okay?" I heard someone ask. I turned around and saw Amal standing there, holding his briefcase. He looked to be in his early thirties and was slim, tallish, and wore thin wire-framed glasses.

"I'm fine," I said quickly, wiping my tears away. "I was just looking at the view."

"Are you sure?" he asked.

The elevator beeped. His fellow doctors were holding the door for him.

"Yes, I'm fine."

He got in the elevator and I watched him and the other doctors disappear behind the closing doors.

I put my face in my hands and leaned against the cold glass, thinking of poor Josie hooked up to powerful painkillers, with burns all over her body. The elevator doors beeped again, and I heard footsteps coming toward me, then felt a hand on my shoulder.

"She is going to be all right. I promise."

I was surprised to see Amal. "I thought you were on your way home."

"I was, but I just wanted to come back and check on you."

He led me over to a green vinyl bench and we sat down. "Josie's in good hands," he said. "We're going to take good care of her, but you need to take care of yourself. You need to get some rest and eat."

This doctor had been on his way home after a long day at work but had taken the slow, crowded elevator back up to the seventh floor so that he could help ease the mental anguish of a worried, exhausted, scared-out-of-her-mind mother. As the days went by, my fondness for Amal grew. He had a quiet confidence about him and I could tell he was a favorite among the nurses, always asking them for their input.

I had never spent time in a hospital other than to have babies. Now, as I kept watch over Josie, I was witnessing human beings at their very best. Every day I watched the brilliant doctors and nurses of Johns Hopkins, with whom I was bonding, take care of sick children. There was one little girl, age seven, who was in the PICU because she chewed her fingers—was literally chewing her fingers off. Her room was connected to Josie's, separated by a glass sliding door. Her mother, young and pretty with short, blonde hair, kept the door closed and the curtain drawn most of the time. Sometimes the nurses opened it and I saw the mother crying softly. I could tell she had been to the PICU many times before.

For a day or two Josie and I had a roommate. His name was Jerome. He was thirteen years old and was mentally and physically disabled. I could see the outline of his deformed legs under the white sheets of his bed and he would situate his body so that he could stare at Josie and me all day. One afternoon I had gotten tired of the staring and closed the curtain.

I asked the nurse on duty where his mother was. She explained to me as I helped her make Josie's bed that his mother would often drop him off for days at a time; this was her idea of babysitting.

After we finished making the bed I opened the curtain and moved my chair so that I was next to him. "Her name's Josie," I said, as he stared at her.

"I like the little baby. Is she okay?"

"Yes, she's going to be fine."

Late that afternoon, on day number six, Josie and I had to leave the room to meet with the physical therapist. As I was walking down the hall pushing Josie's bed, I heard Jerome cry out.

"Please don't take the little baby. Please come back."

I ran back to him and told him we'd only be gone for a half hour. I watched his eyes fill up with tears. "When we come back I'll sit next to you and I'll turn Josie's bed around so that you can see her better," I said.

I felt lucky compared to most of these people. Josie was healing and would soon be going home. They had illnesses from which they would probably never recover.

In the beginning, I never left Josie's bedside. Sometimes I sat in the chair by her bed and let my eyes close as the soft ticking of the monitors lulled me to sleep. One night, when the chair got uncomfortable, I lay down on the floor using my thick, gray cable sweater as a pillow. Amy walked in and saw me. She immediately snapped on rubber gloves and grabbed a garbage bag.

"Are you crazy?" she said, walking toward me. "That floor is filthy." She told me to put the sweater in the garbage bag and take it straight to the dry cleaners. "Wash your hands and, whatever you do, don't touch the sweater."

I got up and dropped the sweater into the garbage bag.

"I just wanted to lie down for a few minutes. The floor is totally clean," I said, pointing to the spotless, white floor that smelled of antiseptic.

Amy opened my eyes to a world I never knew existed. She told me that hospitals were dirty and could be dangerous. "There are germs everywhere and if they get into a patient it can be deadly," she told me. "Not even the most powerful antiseptics can kill them."

I had never heard of hospital-acquired infections or that they kill tens of thousands of patients per year. After she left the room, as I sat there in my chair that I had rubbed down with antiseptic wipes, I wondered why she would say that hospitals were dangerous places. Not Hopkins, I told myself.

After the nurses had enough of seeing me slumped in a chair, and realizing that I did not want to leave Josie's side, they told me about a place, not far away, where I could get a few hours of real sleep.

"There's a room on the ninth floor where there are foldout cots. It's really reserved for mothers of terminally ill patients, but I think there might be an extra cot," one of the nurses said as she handed me a key.

Late at night when I was certain that Josie was comfortable and sleeping soundly, I took the elevator up to the ninth floor, a floor that was almost completely deserted, with no patients and no doctors, just long winding hallways with closed doors. Sometimes I saw a janitor's bucket and mop leaning at one of the doors. It was silent and creepy, ghost-like.

Before stepping out of the elevator I poked my head out, looking both ways to make sure there was no one lurking, and then ran as fast as I could to the locked door that the nurse had described, with the key poised in my hand. I jammed the key in and turned it, opening and then shutting the door quietly behind me. I was safe, in a softly lit room filled with other mothers sleeping soundly on fold-out beds, privacy curtains drawn around each little pod.

There was a bathroom with showers and lockers. I brushed my teeth, washed my face, and tiptoed toward an empty pod. On the table beneath the window lay a guest journal. I picked it up and began reading the stories of the sleeping mothers.

Many were far from home, writing in their native language. Some could barely write at all. Their children were deathly ill, with brain tumors, cancer, sickle-cell anemia, or other rare disorders, and the parents had brought them to Hopkins with hopes of them being healed and going home.

I looked at the pen lying on the table and thought of writing an entry, but what would I say? *My daughter's doing great. I'm so excited. We're going home soon.* My story did not belong with theirs.

I never met any of the mothers. I was always in late and out early, but I felt connected to them as we lay in our beds, our separate worlds, all wanting the same thing: our child to get better. For now, though, we'd take a few hours of sleep. I closed my eyes, realizing how lucky I was, and I promised myself that when I got out of here I would come back and do something for these mothers.

4

It was day number nine when the nurse on duty told me that Josie was going to be moved downstairs to the step-down unit. I immediately went to Amal and pleaded with him to let Josie stay where she was. I wanted him and the nurses there to keep taking care of her.

He explained to me that the PICU was almost over capacity and that Josie was well enough to be moved.

"She'll be fine on the sixth floor," he told me.

That night, two nurses escorted Josie and me down the elevator to our new home on the sixth floor.

"No one has ever been sent back up," one of them told me.

Every day I wrote in my journal, keeping track of each procedure and writing down the name of every doctor, every nurse, and every medication. The writing helped. It made me feel as if I were being productive, as if I had some sort of control over this situation in which, in reality, I was utterly helpless.

The medication I was most concerned with was the morphine. Morphine, as I learned, is a powerful narcotic that suppresses brain activity and decreases the patient's level of consciousness, which, in turn, decreases the level of pain. When too much morphine is administered, the brain often checks out and the signals from the brain that tell the lungs to keep working don't get sent, causing the patient to suffocate. I watched closely to see when and how often her morphine button was pushed. I became concerned one day when we were preparing to make a trip down the hall to the physical therapist's office. Josie was resting peacefully but, as we started our journey, the nurse pushed the pain button. Why was Josie getting more of this drug pumped into her little body when she was sound asleep and obviously not in pain? Why couldn't we let her wake up a little, and if she seemed uncomfortable, then we could give her some relief? Or perhaps we could start a slow wean.

I didn't know this nurse very well, and as we walked down the hall together I tried to think of a way to ask if we could back off the pain button, without coming off as a know-it-all, high-maintenance mother. Or perhaps I should just keep my mouth shut. This woman was a registered nurse. She had gone to school to learn about this stuff. Who was I to question her? I wanted to stay on her good side. And so, as we pushed Josie's bed down the hall, I struck up a conversation.

"What is morphine, exactly?" I asked.

"It's just a really strong painkiller," she said matter of factly.

"How often do you push the button?" I asked hesitantly.

"You can push it whenever she seems uncomfortable, or every few hours."

I asked her if there was anything wrong with pushing it less often or perhaps lowering the dosage if she didn't seem to be in pain.

"Sure," she said. "We can do that."

The constant button pushing subsided, and at each shift change, in which I was now a firm participant, we discussed lowering the morphine dose. Eventually Josie was taken off the powerful drug and given methadone, similar to morphine but much weaker. Josie was beginning to wake up.

It was day ten. Josie was fully awake and eating the pear slices that I was feeding her one by one when we were visited by the detective who had investigated our case. He was a friendly young man in his early thirties, and after he inquired about Josie's progress and made a bit of small talk, I began wondering why he had come to see me. I opened a tin of cookies that I had brought for the nurses and offered them to him. He reached for one as he explained to me that our water heater had been set at the appropriate 120 degrees, but that the actual temperature of the water that came out of that one particular tub faucet was thirty degrees hotter. "It appears that the bushing, which is part of the heat panel, is faulty," he told me.

"What are you saying?" I asked.

"I'm saying that if your water heater setting had been working properly the setting would have read 150 degrees and you would have turned it down to 120. At 120 she would not be here."

Chuck happened to be in the room. I turned to him and asked him what he thought.

"He's right. She definitely wouldn't have needed to be here this long, if at all."

"What are you suggesting?" I asked the detective.

"That you talk to a lawyer."

Chuck scribbled something on a piece of paper and handed it to me. It had a number on it. "Call this man," he said. "He works at a law firm that specializes in product liability. Tell him you're a friend of mine."

I stared at the scrap of paper and put it in my pocket. I had so much to be thankful for. Josie had finished her plate of pears. We would deal with the water heater issue later. I thanked the detective for the information.

That afternoon Tony came by after work. Chuck talked to him about the need to find a lawyer sooner rather than later. A meeting was set up the following day in the waiting room at Hopkins. Meanwhile, the lawyer sent an engineer to the house to do a thorough investigation.

Josie was doing well but had been suffering from an upset stomach and diarrhea. She was checked for an infection, but the tests showed there wasn't one. After a day or two her stomach had settled.

The next day, Tony met the lawyer in the waiting room. Josie was eating, gobbling up everything in sight, and keeping it down. I did not want to leave her, so Tony brought the lawyer back to meet me. He was a nice man, with brown hair and gray sideburns, and he explained that his engineers had found a faulty bushing piece just as the detective had suspected. He thought we had a solid case against the water heater company and wanted to move ahead.

While it was a relief to know what had happened, the situation didn't feel right. We were thankful Josie was doing so well. That was enough; we had all we wanted. We told the lawyer we needed to think about it, and that we hoped to be home soon and could talk then.

That day Josie ate everything on her plate.

* * *

The afternoon of roughly day fourteen, Chuck told Tony and me that he thought Josie would be ready to go home soon. Her wounds no longer needed to be covered in gauze. They had healed well enough to need only a steady influx of Bacitracin. A Thursday discharge was set up, three days from now. We were ecstatic.

Tony and I had talked earlier about wanting to stay involved with the good people at Hopkins, especially Chuck. The patient-doctor relationship had turned into a true friendship. Now seemed like the perfect time to ask him if we could help him raise money for his trauma unit.

"That'd be great," he said, slapping Tony on the back as if they were old college buddies. He invited us to his annual fund-raiser, a chili cook-off. "I love to cook when I'm not at the hospital, and chili is one of my specialties."

We told him we wanted to make a donation and do whatever else he needed us to do. We wanted to stay involved with Hopkins.

While they continued to talk, I sprung into action. I called my mother to tell her we'd be bringing Josie home in three days and suggested that she and the children start planning a welcome home party for her. She told me they had been making posters and cards all week. I called the physical therapist and made an appointment for Josie the following Monday. Josie's homecoming was going to be the happiest day of my life.

The next day, I began noticing that every time someone walked by with a drink Josie would cry for it. I asked the nurse on duty if she could have some water. "No, only ice chips," she said.

I suggested hooking her up to an IV. "She seems thirsty." Again I was turned down.

"She's fine. I don't want her stomach to get upset again," the nurse said.

I filled a cup with ice chips and fed them to Josie slowly throughout the day. She sucked on the chips while I wiped up the melted ice that dripped down her chin.

Later that afternoon, Chuck came in to say hello and to check on Josie. He suggested that he take out her central line. He explained to us that the only reason to keep it in was if she needed medication quickly, and that was highly unlikely. "At this point the IV site is really just a place where an infection might pop up," he explained.

And so he took it out and there she was, free of wires, free of tubes. I could pick her up. It had been two long weeks since I had held her in my arms. She was wearing one of her brother's T-shirts, which hung on her like a long dress. Her legs wrapped around me while her feet dangled beneath the white shirt. She nestled her tired head under my chin.

I had bought Chuck a thank-you present. As I held Josie I reached into my bag and handed him the hardback copy of *Corelli's Mandolin*. Inside, I had inscribed these words:

Dear Chuck,
> Thank you for making us all better.
>> Much love,
>> Josie and the Kings

I walked across the hall to find Amy. I wanted her to finally see Josie awake and well, in my arms and heading home.

I thanked her for all she had done for Josie and for me, and told her that if she was ever having a bad day to remember how happy she made us. She put one hand on my shoulder and ran the other hand along Josie's back. She smiled and told me she was happy we were going home.

It was approaching Josie's bedtime and I helped the nurse on duty give her a bath. As I dribbled water over her head she began sucking on the washcloth. I ran my hand down her naked back. She seemed so thin, thinner than yesterday, thinner than I had ever seen her. I told myself it was because she didn't have clothes on and I laid her down in bed. But something wasn't right. Her color seemed different, paler. Her eyes looked empty, as if she were going to pass out. I told myself it was because she was tired. I stepped back and looked at her. No, something wasn't right.

I asked the nurse if she could take a look and if perhaps we could call a doctor.

"She's fine. Her vitals are fine. Sometimes kids get like this when they've been here for a while. She's just tired," she said, glancing at me before looking back at her computer screen.

I tried to convince myself that the nurse was right, that Josie was just tired, but I couldn't. I asked another nurse if she could take a look.

"She's fine," the second nurse told me. "Go home and get some sleep."

And so I did. I left Josie, telling myself that these nurses were the best. They knew what they were doing. I called two times during the night. Each time I was told that Josie was fine.

*   *   *

Tony left early the next morning for a business trip in California. Josie would be home soon and we had both agreed that he should go see his clients. He would be home by Thursday, the same day Josie would be coming home.

He scraped the ice from my windshield as I turned the ignition on to warm up the car. The two of us stood in the driveway at 5 a.m. that freezing February morning. The children and my mother were inside the old farmhouse sleeping soundly. Soon they would wake up and Big Rel would make them a hearty breakfast, probably oatmeal with fried eggs and bacon all mixed up together—something that would "stick to your ribs and give you energy all day," as she used to tell us when we were kids. I was sure Jack, Relly, and Eva would turn their noses up at it and wonder where their Frosted Flakes and Toaster Strudel were.

Tony wrapped his arms around me. As a married couple and as parents we had been lucky, never being faced with any sort of major adversity or tragedy. Josie being hurt and in the hospital was the worst thing that had ever happened to us and to our family. I was grateful to him for his strength, his steadiness. He calmed my nerves.

"We're on the home stretch," he said. "We're almost there. The next time I see you, Josie will be home. We'll all be together." In the freezing cold, I felt warm against him.

We got in our cars and I followed him down I-83 until he stuck his arm out the window and waved to me as he turned off toward the airport. I felt a strange sort of elation as I drove down Fayette Street to the hospital. Perhaps it was the type of happiness that one can feel only if danger or death has knocked on the door and then walked away. I couldn't wait to see Josie and scoop her up in my arms again. I couldn't wait to bring her home and have our family back the way it was supposed to be, together again.

It was 5:30 a.m. I walked in, said good morning to everyone, and gave the nurse on duty a muffin that I had picked up. I went to Josie's bed and was shocked at how horrible she looked. She was unresponsive, her eyes half open. I ran out into the hall and screamed for help. I saw the team of doctors starting their rounds and called to them to look at Josie. They told me they had a few other patients to see first.

I had always tried to be a low-maintenance parent, but this time I was scared, really scared, and I was not going to sit quietly and wait for our turn. I ran down to the end of the hall and pleaded with them to come now.

They followed me back to her room. I asked them to let her drink something and they allowed it. Josie gulped down nearly a liter of Gatorade. They gave her a shot of Narcan, a drug that is used for drug overdoses, primarily morphine or methadone. Narcan competes with the brain receptor that accepts the methadone. When the Narcan reaches those receptors the methadone can't make it through that door to the brain. After Josie received the shot of Narcan she immediately began looking better. The problem with Narcan is that it has a very short half-life and can wear off in minutes, thus allowing the methadone to creep back into the brain receptors. They gave her another shot of Narcan and she continued to improve.

She had kept the fluids down and she was more alert, looking at me and at the ABC poster that was hanging on the wall.

"She'll be fine," Chuck told me. I asked him if we could skip the 1:00 p.m. dose of methadone.

"Chuck, she doesn't need it. Look at her. She's clearly not in pain, and she's doing better."

Both he and Milissa agreed with me and issued a verbal order that no more narcotics be given. I was still scared and asked the residents to stay close by just in case I needed them. Tony was in the air on his way to California.

The nurse on duty that morning was named Brenda. I had not seen her around before and had an uneasy feeling about her that I couldn't quite explain, so I asked one of the other nurses about her. She told me Brenda was a traveling nurse, one who came to Hopkins through an agency. Often, when hospitals don't have enough nurses they must either turn patients away or call in a backup from a nursing agency.

As I listened to her explanation I thought to myself, *I don't want a traveling nurse. I want a Hopkins nurse.*

I turned to Chuck and asked him what he thought. "She is a little different," he said. "But these agency nurses are pretty darn good." He told me not to worry and walked out of the room just as Brenda returned.

Soon after, a man and a woman wearing white coats walked over to Josie's bed. They looked at the monitors, read her charts, and put a stethoscope to her chest. They told me they were from the pain management team. I told them they were not needed and that Josie would not be receiving pain medication today. Dr. Paidas had given orders.

"Yes, we know," they said. "We just wanted to check on her."

They left the room and I watched them through the glass

window as they stood in the hall talking, writing on their clipboards and looking at Josie through the window.

I decided that I wouldn't worry about Brenda or the pain management team; I had work to do. Josie was looking good, and I was going to begin my routine of rubbing Bacitracin on her hands and feet. I asked Brenda if she could hand me some sterile gloves and a tube of Bacitracin.

"I can't do that, I'm getting ready to take my break," she told me.

"I don't need you to help me. I just need the gloves and ointment, or maybe you can just show me which cabinet they're in?" I pleaded.

She threw twenty tiny tubes of ointment onto Josie's bed and walked out of the room. Amy had seen the transaction and saw me struggling with the sterile gloves and small slippery tubes. She came over, opened the tubes, and squirted the ointment onto my gloved hands.

"Don't worry. She's probably just in a bad mood," she said.

At 1:00 p.m. Brenda walked over with a syringe of methadone.

I asked her what she was doing and told her that Dr. Paidas had given orders for Josie not to receive more methadone. "Don't give it to her," I said as she neared Josie's bed.

"The orders have been changed," she responded.

Something didn't seem right. Why were the orders changed? Should I knock the drug out of her hands and scream for help? Was I missing something? *Stop, slow down,* I told myself. I am at Johns Hopkins, the best hospital in the country. These doctors and nurses are the smartest. They know more than I do. They must have changed the orders for a reason, a good reason. They know what they are doing. I moved aside and stood there as Brenda squirted the drug into Josie's mouth. I continued rubbing ointment on her feet.

"Look, a crocodile tear," Amy said. I looked and there it was, one single tear sliding down Josie's cheek. I wiped it away, thinking to myself how strange it was that in the two weeks since Josie and I had been in the hospital this was the very first tear I had seen.

I began taking off my gloves and cleaning up, but when I looked back at Josie I stopped dead in my tracks. Her eyes had rolled back in her head. "Josie? Josie!" I shook her. She was not responding. I screamed for help. Amy screamed for help and started pushing buttons on the monitors.

"Look at her! Look at her! Someone help!" I screamed.

A dozen nurses and doctors raced to her bed with metal tables and trays and equipment. I felt myself being led out of the room and into the hall, and I felt someone standing next to me, patting my arm. I stood there looking through the glass but I couldn't see Josie. I could only see the backs of white coats and blue scrubs as doctors and nurses surrounded her bed. I wanted to run back to Josie, to comfort her, to tell her everything was going to be all right. I wanted to scoop her up in my arms and run home as fast as I could, but I couldn't. I was paralyzed with fear and dread. I watched Amal Murarka. He raised his hands to the monitors and screamed, "What the hell happened here?"

Breathe, I told myself. Breathe.

They put me in a small, windowless room. A chaplain stood quietly in the corner and I wondered why he was there. My mother raced in. I sank into a chair and put my head on the table. She sat down next to me and put her arms around me. I got up and felt the need to put my face on something cold. I had to put my face on the floor. I lay down next to the table. My head was spinning and my hands tingled. The coolness felt good on my face. Why was the chaplain in here? *No,* Josie was *not* going to die, and we did *not* need him. We were in the best hospital in the world. This was science and technology at its best, and we *were* going home! I got up off the floor. I felt dizzy. I sat next to my mother and laid my head on her lap.

"She's going to be all right, isn't she?"

"Yes, everything is going to be just fine," she said, running her fingers through my hair as my tears silently trickled onto her lap. The chaplain stayed in the corner. His head was bowed. I could hear him mumbling a prayer. Tony's plane was touching down in California.

I don't remember how much time went by before they let me see Josie. They took me up the back steps, back up to the PICU. I walked into the room and saw her lying there, hooked up to machines. I looked at Chuck and the nurses that were standing around her bed and, with all of the conviction and strength that I could find in my heart, I held back my urge to scream at them at the top of my lungs. I said calmly, "*You* did this to her. Now *you've* got to fix her! I don't care what it takes or how much money it'll cost. *Just fix her.*"

No one said a word. I walked over to Josie. She had a breathing tube down her throat and tubes coming out of every part of her body. There was dried blood on the sheet. Her leg was black and blue and partly covered with a bandage.

I looked at Chuck. "What have you done to her?" I demanded.

He told me she had had a cardiac arrest. "They couldn't get the medications through her veins." He paused. "They had to go through the bone in her leg."

I stood looking at Josie in horror. He told me we needed to pray. The others walked by me and some of them reached out and touched my shoulder. They left me standing there alone, with my daughter hooked up to a bunch of machines. Were they giving me a moment alone to be with God and ask for His help? Because that was not going to work. They needed to get back in here and get to work. They needed to fix what they had done.

By this time my father had come down to the hospital. He had reached Tony on his cell as he was walking into his San Francisco office. He handed the phone to me and I told him he needed to come home.

"What do you mean?" he asked. "Josie's all right isn't she?" I could hear the panic in his voice. I couldn't tell him the truth. I couldn't bear to make him sit on the plane knowing that Josie had had a cardiac arrest. So I lied.

"Yes, she'll be fine. Just come home," I paused. "Now."

I sat by Josie watching the pulse of her heartbeat on the monitor. I watched her eyelids, waiting for a flutter. I held her hand, waiting for a squeeze. I waited for hours, but nothing came.

Tony arrived at 6:00 p.m. He rushed to her bed and stared, speechless, taking in the horrible sight of her.

"She had a cardiac arrest," I told him. "She's going to be all right. She's going to be fine."

The news that something had gone terribly wrong at the

hospital started spreading. Family and friends began flying and driving to Baltimore from California, Boston, and Virginia.

Hours passed. Tony and I sat on either side of Josie's bed, waiting for her to wake up. I stood and went into the little windowless room that had become our own private waiting room. It was 1:00 a.m and Margaret, my sister, was sitting there. I lay down to put my face against the cool floor. She got two pillows and a blanket and lay next to me. She wrapped her arms around me and told me everything was going to be all right. There was nothing else she could possibly say. I wanted to close my eyes and leave this horrible nightmare. I walked back into Josie's room and laid my head on her bed and held her hand, waiting, praying for a squeeze.

As my family tried to connect the dots to find what precisely had gone wrong they inundated Dr. Paidas, Dr. McKee, and any doctor or nurse who walked down the hall with questions. "What happened? She was fine just yesterday. She was on her way home." "How could she have had a cardiac arrest?" "She's going to be all right, isn't she?"

Within hours of Josie's cardiac arrest Hopkins began scrambling to collect information. Blood cultures were sent to the lab for testing as they searched for signs of a massive infection. They were searching for something to blame other than themselves. It had to be the fault of the imperfect human body. At Chuck's suggestion we had a meeting, all of us: Tony, my parents and my sister, Milissa, Amal, some nurses, and myself.

"Should we meet in the conference room?" Chuck suggested.

"No, I will not leave Josie. We'll have the meeting in her room," I said.

Chairs were brought in and a circle was formed to the side of Josie's bed, which Tony and I sat next to. Chuck began the meeting explaining to us that they did not know what had gone wrong and that she had probably acquired some sort of massive, fast-moving infection, perhaps sepsis.

I looked at my family; some had their arms folded across their chests, some were sitting on the edge of their seats as they listened to Chuck and others explain, in complicated medical terms, why Josie was on the brink of death.

"No, that's wrong Chuck. You're all wrong," I blurted out. Everyone turned to look at me. "I was there. I saw it all happening." I stood up. "She was thirsty and you gave her methadone. She shouldn't have gotten the methadone. It was the drugs and dehydration. And you all know it."

The head of the PICU interjected that they would wait for the results of the blood cultures, that there would be an investigation, and that it could take weeks to determine why she had the cardiac arrest.

As I sat down I realized that the wedge had been placed between me and the doctors and nurses with whom I had once been friends.

I looked at Josie's body. None of what they said or what I said mattered. It was all pointless, a waste. I didn't want an explanation. I wanted a miracle.

The neurologists came at 8:00 a.m. the next morning. There were four of them, each carrying a black case. They suggested that the family wait in the hall.

"But I don't want to wait in the hall," I said. "I want to stay here with Josie."

They looked at Tony. "It would be better if you leave while we examine her."

Tony and I stood in the hall leaning against the wall. We didn't say much. We just waited. My old nurse friends from the weeks before walked past us. I expected them to stop, say hello, tell me that Josie was going to be fine. But they didn't. They couldn't even look at me. Our relationship had become toxic.

When the examination was over, we went back in and sat next to Josie. I held her small hand and stared at her closed eyes. I could feel the neurologists' eyes on me. I didn't want to look at them. I didn't want to hear them. I wanted them to get out of her room.

They told us that Josie was brain dead. Tony put his head in his hands.

"What does that mean?" I asked.

"It means she will not live. Her organs are slowly beginning to shut down. Her liver is no longer functioning. At this point it's just a matter of time before her heart stops beating."

I looked at her tiny body. How could they have done this to her? She had been so thirsty. I saw it happening, the dehydration getting worse and worse and then the methadone, that horrible drug. It was as if she had run a marathon and then a bottle of vodka had been forced down her throat.

"No, please, please don't say that." I let go of Josie's hand and walked around her bed. I stood in front of them. "Look, what about a transplant of some sort? What about brain surgery or something? I know you can make her better," I pleaded. They shook their heads. "Please, you have to help her. Please, don't let this happen. What about a miracle?"

I begged, wiping the tears from my face. "There'll be a miracle."

They said there would be no miracle. There was nothing anyone could do. They snapped their black cases shut and filed out of the room.

I sat down and all of a sudden it hit me head on. It was crystal clear. There *was* a God. How could something so outrageously out of this world, so incomprehensibly horrible, possibly happen? There was no way that this could be happening by natural causes. Some powerful force was controlling this situation and making it more and more unbelievable. The accident, the water heater, the thirst, the methadone, no one listening to me. She didn't stand a chance. This God was going to take her no matter what.

I put my head on Josie's bed and held her motionless hand. I could hear people coming in and whispering. I could not move.

My parents brought Jack, Relly, and Eva down to the hospital. Monica, the fast-talking patient-service coordinator, gave us a quick rundown on preparing young children for how to say good-bye to a sibling. The children walked in and Tony and I hugged them. We went into Josie's room and they looked at her lying there. We explained to them that Josie was going to heaven soon and that they would not see her ever again. We needed to say good-bye now. They looked at her and then at the machines and then at their aunts and uncles. I asked them if they wanted to kiss her good-bye.

Jack said no. Relly said no. Eva said no. My mother took them home.

I look back at those moments and am sorry that I did not think more clearly. I should have asked everyone to leave. It should have just been the six of us in that room. We should have spent more time making the children feel comfortable. They were too confused with all of their aunts and uncles in the room, wondering why everyone was at the hospital. They were six, five, and three, too young to understand.

I wish I had made it better for them. I wish they had kissed her good-bye.

Maybe we should have never let them come down to the hospital in the first place. What a horrible way for them to see their little sister. I hope that they don't remember her like that, hooked up to machines, with a tube down her throat. I hope they remember her full of life and dancing to the Barney song. What was the point of saying good-bye anyway?

We wanted Amal to be the doctor to take Josie off life support. He had healed Josie's wounds. And we wanted Amy to be there with us. They had been with us from the beginning.

Although neither Tony nor I were overly religious we had baptized the other three children and had planned on baptizing Josie in the spring. Tom, a close friend who was a minister, baptized her as we stood by her side. He trickled the water over her forehead. I watched, hoping for her to magically wake up and cry, annoyed that cold water was being poured on her head. I wiped the water off of her motionless face. Tony and I were each given a rocking chair. We sat side by side and Tom stood behind us. Amal turned off the switches and removed the tubes. I leaned over to pick her up and carried her to the rocking chair. I held her, and then Tony held her. Amal got up and listened to her heart. It was still beating. Slowly.

I asked Tom to say something, anything.

I held her, and then Tony and I held her together, Tony's arm around me and the other draped under mine as we clung to her and to each other. The minutes ticked by. Amal laid the stethoscope on her chest again. He looked at us and nodded. She died in our arms and my heart exploded into a million pieces.

I looked out the window, which had turned orange from the setting sun. Large snowflakes began falling slowly from the clouds above, and the fiery sky turned them a pale shade of pink, like nothing I had seen before.

5

In forty-eight hours we had gone from planning a welcome home celebration to planning a funeral. God, or whoever created us, was very clever when He programmed into our systems a mechanism called shock. Shock is a fabulous narcotic. It can block the brain from sending damaging information to the heart and soul. It is a mechanism that protects us from feeling excruciating pain. As in a car crash, the impact takes place but at some point in time the brain blacks out. The body feels no pain as bones break and flesh is ripped apart.

Most researchers agree that in the face of crippling fear, pain, or grief, the body releases endorphins. When these endorphins connect to the receptors in our brain a sense of numbness is created, preventing the body from being overwhelmed, making it so that the mind is unable to process the trauma all at once. The only problem with shock is that it does not last forever. Psychologists say that shock is the first stage of the grieving process and can last anywhere from a few days to a few weeks, after which time the endorphin levels subside and the brain shifts the event into perspective. We are faced with the broken bones, the torn flesh, and the shattered heart.

I had never needed sleeping pills or antidepressants, and I never understood why people did. I thought all problems could be solved with a good old-fashioned rush of endorphins: a run in the woods and a dose of fresh air.

Now, every evening my father came to me and I held out my hand and swallowed the little pink pill he offered. I walked downstairs where all of the family was gathered and sat on the sofa. Sometimes Tony sat beside me and put his arm around me. I listened to the voices, the sounds of people coming and going, bringing more flowers, more food, and more gifts for the children. I watched the children rip through the wrapping as if it was Christmas morning, as if the gifts would magically trick them into thinking everything was all right.

Eva climbed onto my lap with her new doll. I held her and tried to keep my eyes open as the sleeping pill started working and my head wobbled around on my neck. I fell into a soft, drug-induced haze. Someone reached down to take Eva from me. Tony led me up the stairs and laid me down in bed, pulling the covers over me. He lay next to me and I closed my eyes and let the darkness take me away.

With the help of the drug, I was at peace, and sometimes I dreamed about Josie. I dreamed that she was running toward me in the field behind our house. I dreamed that she was in her car seat and I was handing her a Gatorade. She was better, and I was happy.

But like shock, sleep ends and you wake up. In those waking moments the dream faded, the haze lifted, and I realized that Josie was not in her crib. It was as if a knife were plunging into my heart and the pain I felt was excruciating. Usually this happened to me in the early morning hours. In my misery I thought about sneaking up to my parents' room to rifle through their belongings until I found what I needed: the bottle of sleeping pills.

Parents should not have to plan a funeral for their child. Seeing we were paralyzed with grief, my father took over. My sister Margaret worked on a eulogy. Tony's sister, Susan, and older brother, Jay, designed and printed cards. My mother-in-law, Carol, arranged for all the food, and my mother started a notebook and file box where all the letters and gifts were organized for us to see at some later date. The snow was shoveled and there was constant sledding and entertainment for Jack, Relly, and Eva.

Our daughter's funeral was being planned and all we did was nod our heads at my father as he selected hymns and prayers. Sometimes he brought Tony and me into the living room and closed the door. We sat on the sofa and listened to him as he ever so gently read us a draft of what was going to be submitted to the obituary section. We listened as he ever so gently brought up the subject of cremation. There were some decisions that only we could make.

I don't remember much about the service. I don't remember what songs were sung or what prayers were read. I don't remember if the children sat quietly or fidgeted. The images in my mind are hazy and blurred, including the ones of Margaret standing before the congregation and delivering the eulogy that she had written: "Josie, when you clap your hands in heaven there will be thunder. When you blow a kiss, fresh snow will fall on the Rocky Mountains, and your father will enjoy a powder day . . ."

I do remember standing outside the church after the service. My brother Mac put his arm around my shoulder, squeezing me tightly. I held on to Relly's hand. Jack and Eva stood next to Tony. There was silence except for the church bells, which rang and rang. Everyone looked at us with their heads bowed, waiting for something to happen. I wanted them to leave and stop looking at us. I wanted the ringing to stop.

"Can we go home now?" I asked my brother.

He took my hand and we walked through the crowd toward the car. The people parted like the Red Sea. Hands reached out to touch us. The Suburban seemed miles away and my legs felt shaky. We climbed in and the doors closed softly.

I looked out the window as the car pulled away and searched the crowd for the Hopkins doctors and nurses. There was one thing I could see with clarity that day, one thing I knew I needed to have happen: they had to come to the house. I didn't care about seeing family or friends. I wanted only to see the people who were responsible for this.

I could have wanted them there because they were good doctors and nurses and had become my friends; they never meant to hurt Josie and I knew they, too, were sad and in pain. In reality there was a part of me that wanted them there only to make their pain worse. I wanted them to see Josie's grandparents, who had lost their granddaughter, and Josie's aunts and uncles, who no longer had a niece. And most of all I wanted them to see Josie's siblings; their little sister had been taken away from them.

They came to our house and I accepted them graciously, making sure they had a plate of food and a drink. I wanted them to see with their own eyes that what they had done was more than a bad day on the job. I wanted them to see our beautiful home, a house whose walls screamed for a big family with children running through it, and I wanted them to realize they had taken it all away.

6

Two weeks after Josie died, Dr. George Dover, the head of the Johns Hopkins Children's Center, and Dr. Lauren Bogue, Josie's pediatrician, came to the house. It was a cold stormy night and they came in dripping with wet umbrellas.

Dr. Dover was a tall portly man with gray hair and a beard. In his late fifties, he was a pediatrician who specialized in hematology. Dr. Bogue was the pediatrician who had cared intimately for all four of our children. Short, with brownish gray hair, she had a kind, motherly way about her. She was the perfect pediatrician. During Josie's stay at Hopkins she often visited us and checked on Josie.

She was the first person from Hopkins to come to us after Josie had her cardiac arrest. She told us what she suspected and what I already knew: Josie should not have had a cardiac arrest. "Don't worry," she had said to Tony and me. "I've already talked to the head of the Children's Center. They're going to get to the bottom of this."

We went into the living room. The two of them sat side by side on the sofa and Tony and I sat in chairs on either side. A fire was burning in the fireplace and a picture of Josie lay on the coffee table. An awkward silence set in.

Dr. Dover began by telling us he was sorry. He had come to us to offer an apology. "Josie should not have died," he said. "I am so sorry." We listened to him as he nervously continued on, using terms like "sentinel event," "root cause analysis," and "morbidity and mortality meetings." "We have a team investigating the case. We will get to the bottom of it and we'll report all of our findings to you."

Report their findings? I didn't care about some investigative committee or what their findings were. I knew what had happened. "Dr. Dover," I said, "Josie died because you all didn't listen, and you being here tonight talking to us, apologizing, doesn't change anything."

I waited for a response, listening to the snap of the fire as the tension rose.

"We know this is difficult," Dr. Bogue said. "We're here because we want you both to know that Hopkins is taking full responsibility."

"Let the investigation move forward," Dr. Dover said. "Give us a few months." He suggested that we talk once a week. He would give us updates on the investigation. I didn't really care about listening to his updates, but I did like the idea of having him on the other end of the phone where he would be forced to listen to my tirades, my raw anger and grief. We set the date for every Friday at 1:00 p.m. Whatever else they said that cold rainy night did not matter to us at the time.

As they were conducting their investigation, we would be assembling the best team of lawyers to destroy them. In my mind there was going to be a bloodbath, and planning it gave me little breaks from my grief. I moved in and out of two emotions: utter and complete sadness and a burning all-consuming anger. In the sadness, the feeling of loss was so great that I could not move. I was frozen completely helpless.

The pain was so intense that sometimes I would ache for some sort of physical pain, a sliced arm, a broken bone, something to take my mind off the pain I felt in my heart.

In my anger I would feel an energy that I couldn't get rid of. It kept me up at night and made me pace back and forth across the room, shaking my head and saying "Why, why, why?" My mind was spinning with all the things I was going to do to make Hopkins feel my pain. I was coming up with a brilliant PR campaign that would destroy them. I would take Hopkins apart brick by brick. They would never forget Josie King.

Happiness, joy, and laughter no longer seemed a part of my genetic makeup. I was a different person now. I felt as though my DNA had changed. It was exhausting.

Not long after Dr. Dover and Dr. Bogue's visit we received a phone call from Hopkins' lead attorney, Rick Kidwell. He explained to us that the investigative team had been selected and that their work was under way. He asked if we would attend a meeting.

"I want the team to do more than analyze records and interview doctors. I want them to hear from you. They need your perspective," he said.

A few days later, Tony and I walked into the famous domed building, past the giant Jesus statue that stood in the center of the building's rotunda, and up the winding staircase into the risk management office. Mr. Kidwell, well over six feet, with graying hair, shook our hands and led us down the hall to the conference room. He introduced us to the members of the team: a surgeon, an ICU doctor, an intensive care doctor, two pediatric nurses, and another risk manager. Josie's death was a sentinel event: an event in which there has been an unexpected outcome resulting in death or serious injury. The team's job was to investigate the case, determine what had gone wrong and why, and come up with a solution to prevent it from happening again. These root cause analysis meetings are mandatory investigations that take place in hospitals around the country whenever there has been a sentinel event.

The conference room was dungeon-like, with gray walls and small windows that were fifteen feet above the floor, barely letting in the light. Mr. Kidwell asked me to tell the group what I had seen at the hospital.

"I began noticing her thirst two days before she had the arrest. I asked the nurse twice if we should give her a drink. The nurse said no. I put her to bed. She didn't look good. I asked for help. I wanted to call the doctor but the nurse told me Josie was fine. I asked if another nurse could look at her and again I was assured that Josie was fine.

"The next morning when I saw Josie I screamed for help. I begged them to let her drink. She drank a liter of fluid. They gave her two doses of Narcan. She was better. All she needed was fluids. She would have been fine. She would have lived, but you gave her methadone when I begged you not to. It was the combination of the two. If she had gotten the methadone and had not been dehydrated she would have lived. If she had been dehydrated and not received the methadone she would have lived. She died from severe dehydration and a methadone overdose. She died because you did not listen to me."

No one said anything.

Mr. Kidwell solemnly thanked us for our time and we left the room. As Tony and I walked down the hall I remembered something in my coat pocket and told him I'd be right back. I ran back to the conference room and knocked on the door. I could hear them talking. Mr. Kidwell opened the door, surprised to see me. "I forgot something," I said, walking past him. I handed each person a picture of Josie. "This is for you, to remind you that this is more than just a case study."

We were unaware that this was the first time, not only in the history of Hopkins but possibly in the history of health care, that a family had been invited to attend a root cause analysis meeting. Years later, Rick Kidwell's approach to including the family would be slowly adopted in other health care institutions around the country.

While Hopkins investigated Josie's death, Tony and I began interviewing lawyers. We met with a large prestigious law firm in Washington, DC, that specialized in medical malpractice. Tony's father, who was a lawyer, had spoken to them a number of times about Josie's case. We drove to Washington to meet with them and were escorted to a large conference room. The large shiny table was surrounded by serious-looking men and women in suits. They had paper and glasses of water in front of them. They stood up when we came in and sat down when we were seated. They listened. They asked questions. They scribbled notes and sipped their water. They explained how they would handle the case, who would make up the various teams, and to what extent the press would be involved.

I started drifting away from the conversation, falling back into my world without Josie. My anger was fading into sadness. All I wanted was to have her back. I could hear them talking about fees and percentages. I could see them nodding their heads. I concentrated on holding back my tears but I was too tired. The tears slid down my face. I got up and left the room. I wandered around and found myself in front of a refrigerator. I reached in and took a Diet Coke. One of the men from the meeting found me and asked if I was all right.

"I was just thirsty," I said, wiping the tears away and putting the Coke back.

"Oh no, you can have that," he said. "Here let's pour it in a glass for you."

He handed me the drink and took me back to the meeting. They tried not to look at me as I quietly took my seat with my Diet Coke in front of me. The meeting ended and we got in the car and headed back to Baltimore. Tony and his father talked a little bit about the meeting while I sat in the back seat and stared out the window. The ride was mostly silent. I think we all realized that no matter how much of a powerhouse this law firm was, they could not bring Josie back.

Two days later, we met with Paul Bekman, a partner at Salsbury, Clements, Bekman, Marder and Adkins LLC, a local outfit whose office was two miles down the road from Hopkins. He told us that he and Rick Kidwell, the Hopkins' lead attorney, were acquaintances and had tried a few cases together. "Rick Kidwell is a good and fair man," he said. I sat, looking at the golf pictures that hung on the walls of his office, wondering, *Where's the big fancy conference room? Where are the teams of experts? Why is he not talking about getting the press involved? Why is he telling us what a great guy Rick Kidwell is? This man clearly is not out for blood.*

After three minutes of listening to him and Tony's father talk about golf courses it became apparent to me that Paul was not our guy. We needed that powerhouse law firm down in Washington, DC. They would be the ones to take us to war, not this friend of Kidwell's.

Days later and after much discussion, my father and Tony's father came to Tony and me with their recommendation. They had done some research on Paul Bekman and thought he was our guy. Their argument was that Hopkins was extremely powerful, and that it was better to go with someone that Hopkins already had a relationship with and respect for. Tony agreed with them.

I was too sad and tired to argue.

7

A few weeks after Josie died, Tony called me from work and told me he was going to the funeral home. He had to pick up her ashes. I felt my stomach sink, not wanting to face what they had done to her body.

I hung up the phone and imagined Tony going to the funeral home, walking up to the counter, and picking up her ashes, just like going to the dry cleaners. Would he put them in the front seat or the back seat? I knew I should call him and offer to go with him but I was too stuck in my own pain to pick up the phone.

I slapped together hamburger patties, watching Eva and Relly outside as they jumped on the trampoline. Jack sat at the kitchen table doing his homework and asked when Dad was coming home. I told him that he had an errand to run and would be home later.

"What kind of errand?" he asked.

"I don't know, Jack. Just do your homework," I said as my eyes filled with tears.

"I need help with my math."

"I can help you," I said, as I washed the meat off my hands.

He looked at me as I wiped the tears away. He said he didn't want me to help him. He wanted Dad. I knew Tony would be walking in the door at any minute. My heart started pounding. "I'm really good at math. Let me help you," I said. I stared at the addition problems, thinking to myself, *Don't make me have to explain cremation to the children.* "First we need to sharpen this pencil," I said as I walked to the electric pencil sharpener. I stuck the pencil in the hole and listened to the wood grind. I heard the dogs bark. I watched Relly and Eva hop off the trampoline and run to the driveway.

Tony was home. I wanted to disappear. I wanted Tony to disappear. I wanted it all to disappear.

He walked in with his briefcase slung over his shoulder. He had Eva in one arm and the newspapers I had left in the driveway in the other.

"Dad, I need help with my math," Jack said.

"All right, just let me put my stuff upstairs, and I'll be right down," he answered.

I watched him disappear, the pencil still shoved in the sharpener. I knew what he was going to do. I took the pencil out and blew the dust off. Relly and Eva were playing on the floor with their Polly Pockets. Tony came back down and gave me a weak smile. I handed him the sharpened pencil and walked toward the steps. He asked where I was going. "To the bathroom," I lied.

I knew he had hidden them, and I knew where to look. They would be on the top shelf, behind his ski stuff, with the Skittles and Starbursts that he saved for the kids' chairlift rides. I grabbed a chair and climbed up.

There it was: a tin box. It was not like the kind of tin box that my grandmother gave me when I was a little girl—the kind that was blue and white and filled with rows of butter cookies, the kind that I kept long after all the cookies had been eaten and used to store my mood ring and pukka shell necklace, my prized possessions.

The tin box that I stared at as I stood on the chair with tears streaming down my face was an ugly fake-wood brown. I reached out, took hold of it, and jumped down. I walked into the bedroom, closed the door, and sat on the bed, holding it in my hands.

It was smaller than I would have thought. Smaller than a cookie tin, it was more like the size of a box of chocolates or one that held a special baseball. I had to open it. I could not bear the thought of some mortician's eyes being the last eyes on her.

I carefully pried open the lid, looked in, and saw a white plastic bag tied in a knot. I untwisted the knot and the bag opened. The ashes didn't seem like the ashes left from a campfire. They looked softer and not as dark. I wanted to touch them but I couldn't. Josie wouldn't have wanted me to. She would want me to remember holding her the way I used to.

"Oh, Josie, I'm so sorry." I carefully tied up the bag and closed the lid. I heard the door open and quickly put the tin under the pillow as Tony walked in. He asked me what I was doing. I pulled the pillow away.

"Did you open it?" he asked.

"Yes, did you?"

"No."

"Do you want me to open it for you?" I asked.

He sat down on the bed next to me and I opened it up and handed it to him. He looked in. I could tell he was trying to be strong for me. He looked tired and pale and I wanted to tell him that it was all right to cry. He tied the bag up and put the lid back on.

71

"Where should we keep them? Someone is going to find them if we leave them there," I said.

He sat quietly, thinking. "Let's put them in the little closet with the Christmas ornaments. No one will look for them there and that door is impossible to open."

The closet was accessed by a small two-foot-by-two-foot door at the stairwell landing. It could not be opened without a knife to pry it. Inside, it smelled like candy canes and balsam and was crammed with boxes of ornaments, wrapping paper, a tree stand, Christmas books, and a crèche.

I watched Tony as he carefully opened the crèche that had been wrapped in toilet paper by Eva and Josie just a few months ago and nestled the tin alongside Mary, Joseph, and the wise men. He closed the door, making sure that it could not be opened.

The ashes sat untouched for four months until one day in early May when Tony suggested that perhaps it was time.

"Time for what?" I asked.

"Time to take her ashes to Virginia and bury them," he said.

"Oh, no, let's just leave them with the Christmas ornaments a little longer. Why can't we just leave them there forever? It's cheery and cozy. I don't want them to be in the cold ground so far away from us," I said.

He told me it would be weird and morbid if we left them in the Christmas closet forever. "I've talked to your parents about it. We can go next weekend."

Deep down I knew he was right, that we had to do it. We told the children we were going back to Virginia to see Big Rel and Pop. They were excited for the trip. We decided to let them remain blissfully clueless for a little bit longer. We packed the car and left the key with our neighbors, who promised to take care of Trapper.

As we drove up the gravel driveway to my parents' house, I looked across the field at our old house. The perennial bed that I had planted was bursting with bloom and the tiny Carolina jasmine vine was reaching high above the porch column. The setting sun cast a soft golden glow on the house. If we had never left, Josie would be alive. I wanted the family who had bought our house to get out. I wanted my beautiful life in Virginia back.

My parents were sitting on the front steps when we drove up. The children scrambled out of the car and ran to hug them, begging Big Rel to take them on a golf cart ride.

"I've got it all charged and ready to go," she said, grabbing a bag out of the back of our car. She put her arm around my shoulder and squeezed me as we walked up the blue stone steps to the house. "I know this is hard," she said. "We're going to get through this weekend." She handed each of the children a plastic cup and filled them with pistachios, and then they raced to the golf cart. "Come with us for a ride," she said. My father was fixing Tony a drink and I knew they would soon be engrossed in some work-related conversation.

"No, you all go ahead. I'll stay and unpack," I said, my sadness mounting.

"Come with us," she said. "Let's all be together. You can just sit in the golf cart and we'll go down to the pond. You can cry if you want, and we won't bother you. It'll make you feel better."

I told her to go on. "The children will have more fun without me."

I watched them drive away. I was glad the children were with my mother. They seemed happier without me.

The morning of the burial I woke up and heard the sound of boots softly clumping down the hallway. I heard the front door quietly open and close. I got out of bed and tiptoed to the window, not wanting to wake Tony. I looked out the window and saw my father and Tom, Margaret's husband, wearing their church suits and boots, putting two shovels in the back of the green pickup truck. I stood there as the seconds ticked by and I began to realize what they were going to do. I watched the truck slowly drive down the long driveway and head off toward the church.

I could smell bacon frying and coffee brewing and went into the kitchen. My mother was making pancakes for the children, who were sitting at the counter coloring pictures. I sat next to them and sipped the coffee that she handed me. Relly showed me her picture; it was a balloon floating up into the sky. "It's for Josie," she told me.

"Relly, shut up. You're going to make her cry," Jack said.

"No, Jack, it's okay. I'm not going to cry. Here, let me see."

"They're for when we bury Josie. Big Rel said they can go to heaven with her," Eva said.

I asked Jack to hand me some paper and began to make one myself.

My mother sat with us while we all colored pictures for Josie. I looked over at Relly as she finished her second drawing: a picture of a house with stick figures of each of us and Josie in the air with wings like a bee. Under each figure were our names and under the little bee was Josie's name, each letter completely backward, a mirror image of the word, something I had never seen her do before. I realized that behind that head of blonde hair and that happy face, there was something weighing heavily in her mind as she wrote her sister's name.

They finished their breakfast and hopped off their stools to play with the toys that my mother had stashed in the bunkroom closet.

"How do you think they seem?" I asked as my mother moved to the stool next to me.

"They seem good. They're young and resilient. They're gonna get us all through this," she said.

"We haven't told them anything about the ashes or cremation. How are we supposed to explain that to them?" I asked, as I put my face in my hands.

"I don't think you need to worry about that now. Let's just get through the day. Tomorrow will be better," she said, putting her arm around my shoulder. "Here, drink this." She got up and poured me some of her protein shake. Her goopy mixtures always tasted the same: chalky and fruity, with a variation of whatever new health product she was into that month. "It's got flaxseed oil. It's good for you."

Tony was still asleep, so she poured some coffee for him and handed it to me. I walked down the hall past the old grandfather clock whose faint chimes I had grown up with. I ran a hand down its smooth mahogany side. When I was Relly's age, I used to pretend that a little fairy named Tinkerbell lived inside the clock. I turned the key and opened the door. I put my head in and breathed the old familiar smell of woodsy mustiness, of childhood and magic. The smell of years gone by.

Tony was awake, lying in bed. I handed him the coffee and I climbed in next to him. I showed him the picture that Relly had drawn. "What do you think?" I asked, pointing to Josie's name.

He looked at the picture. "I think there's a lot going around in her head when she thinks of Josie. Maybe that's her way of processing it," he said. "We just need to keep an eye on them. Keep them close by."

The children were dressed in their church clothes and I went outside and pushed Eva around on the tricycle as Jack and Relly fought over a scooter. As we were preparing to load the car, the phone rang inside. My father answered it and then I could see him talking with Tony in the den. Tony walked out the door and whispered in my ear. The neighbors had called. They had found Trapper dead in his dog house that morning.

I don't remember feeling particularly sad. There was just no room in my heart for more pain. Tony and I had bought him in college and he had been with us for as long as we had been together. The children never really paid any attention to him, except for Josie. That was what rattled me that morning. Josie loved him.

We drove to St. Mary's, a pretty little white church in the country outside of Richmond. Reverend John Miller, the preacher, was a kind man who had recently lost his wife to cancer. Tony carried Josie's ashes in the metal tin to Reverend Miller's office as the children and the rest of the family waited by the open grave. Tony handed him the ashes and I handed him a little wooden box. Glued to the lid was the photograph of the children that I had taken the summer before. He left the room to transfer the ashes, came back, and handed the wooden box to Tony. The three of us walked through the cemetery, maneuvering around the gravestones. Reverend Miller put his arm out for me to hold on to and I looked at the gravestones spread all around me. I told him that I hated the word cemetery and that I hated the word graveyard.

"I do, too," he told me, leading me forward. "I call it a church yard. That's what it is. It's a beautiful church yard." We arrived at the small, shallow hole in the ground. Tony handed me the box and I laid it in the hole. The children put their pictures on top of it. Reverend Miller said something— I don't remember what—and we slowly covered the little box with dirt. Reverend Miller knelt down next to Jack, Relly, and Eva and patted the mound with his hands. They looked at him and then knelt next to him and smoothed out the dirt as if they were building a sand castle.

My siblings and parents stepped aside as Tony, the children, and I stood together looking at the mound of dirt. They looked at each other, looked at the playground across the way, and then looked up at us.

"Can we go to the playground now?" Relly asked.

They wiped their hands off on their clothes and raced to the playground, laughing as they jumped over each gravestone, like little ponies. We stared at them in shock, not knowing what to think, and then we looked at each other and laughed. I realized, at that moment on that horrible, horrible day, that just like my mother had said, these three children would pull us all through.

8

Later that month, Tony's mother and sister Susan flew out to Baltimore. They had decided that Tony and I should go away for the night and that they would take care of the children. I wasn't sure about leaving them, but Tony said it would be good for us to get away. He was the one who did all the research whenever we traveled, booking flights, lining up rental cars, picking out hotels. He would even go online and check out menus before suggesting a restaurant.

"It'll be great. I've got it all planned out," he said, trying to convince me to go. He had picked St. Michaels, a charming little town on the Eastern Shore. We'd stay at an inn, have dinner at a cozy restaurant, and go for an early morning bike ride the next day before heading home. "It's just an hour and a half away," he said. "We'll be back in twenty-four hours."

The more I thought about it the more I realized the children were the ones who really needed the break. They would have much more fun hanging out with their awesome grandmother and aunt than having to be with their sad, miserable parents. We packed our bags and put our bikes in the car. As we said good-bye, I noticed that Jack, Relly, and Eva looked the happiest I had seen them since Josie died. Maybe a change of scenery would be good for all of us.

It was late spring, my first spring without Josie, and Maryland was in full bloom. The daffodils and azaleas were bursting with color. We rolled down the windows and looked at the farms as we drove down Maryland's Eastern Shore. The smell of cut grass and the hum of tractors lifted my spirits. I told myself I was not going to think about her.

We checked into the hotel and walked around. The town was charming, just as Tony had said. The shopkeepers had their doors open and across Main Street we could see boats lining the dock. We walked over to look at them before heading to dinner. Tony threw his arm over my shoulder as we crossed the street. An older couple walked by us and smiled. I wondered if they smiled because they thought we were newlyweds, perhaps on a honeymoon. Wouldn't that be nice? A newlywed couple with nothing to think about other than the future. Nothing to plan, aside from exciting careers and starting a family. Perhaps looking at us took them back to younger years as a happy couple embarking on life together. They had no idea what I actually felt like: an old woman with a face like a dried apple.

At dinner, the waitress led us to a table for two next to the window. As she handed us menus and told us the specials, I looked out through the glass and felt the sadness creeping inside of me. My eyes began to sting. I concentrated hard on what she was saying. I stared at the menu. I didn't want to cry. I wanted to forget just for a little bit longer.

I could hear Tony talking to her about the wine list. Even in college, he had an affection for food and wine, especially the California pinots. Being from Sonoma County and having a mother who was a fabulous cook probably had something to do with it.

*   *   *

In Boulder, at the University of Colorado, he lived in a little house on Euclid Avenue with two other guys. The place was a typical college dump: a front porch with beer cans sitting on the railing, and Hacky Sacks, Frisbees, and dirty tennis shoes scattered about. A few kitchen chairs stood in the overgrown grass and mountain bikes cluttered the sidewalk that led to the front steps. A faded Indian batik tapestry hung in the living room and skis were stashed in the corner waiting for the first snowfall. The combined smell of the dirty clothes and spilled beer compelled most visitors to stay on the front porch that looked up to the Flat Iron mountain range.

The only room that might have been acceptable to a mother was the kitchen. Besides the ever-present dirty dishes in the sink, there were always a few perfectly ripened mangoes on the windowsill, knives hanging neatly from the magnetic rack, and spices lined up on the counter next to the stove. In the fridge, tucked behind the Coors and California Coolers, were fresh meats and vegetables. A few pots and pans hung on hooks above the telephone. This was Tony's haven, and by the end of the first semester, most people figured out that the kitchen was the place to be. Good food was to be had. And if you wanted any, you had to help, and that usually meant a little slicing, dicing, and stirring. Of course, cold beer was a part of the deal.

Before Tony, I was happy with a bowl of Grape-Nuts for dinner, but now I was dating a ski racer from northern California, and if he wanted to take me out to a nice restaurant for good food and wine, I was okay with that. His favorite restaurant back then was the Morgul-Bismarck, named after a famous bike route near Boulder.

One night he asked the waiter questions like, "Are the mushrooms for the grilled duck portobellos or chanterelles?" "Would you recommend the 1982 pinot or the chardonnay?" The waiter asked me what I wanted to order but I had not really been focusing on the menu. I asked Tony what he was going to have.

"Grilled duck in the portobello sauce," he said.

I told the waiter I'd have the same.

This thoroughly annoyed Tony and he ordered something else. The waiter poured the wine and as we sipped Tony told me about the vineyard where the wine was from and how he had gone to school with the owner's son. I was from a part of Virginia where grapes and vineyards were as foreign as shad roe and grits were to him.

As he talked I dipped my cloth napkin into my glass of water and then placed it over the wine label. I held it perfectly still until the label was just wet enough, and then I gently peeled it off the green bottle and laid it next to the candle to dry.

I liked my boyfriend from California. I liked hearing about his life in Sonoma County and I liked looking at him from across the table. We didn't talk much about big life decisions or the future, but I could see it: I could see us living in northern California, having lots of children and teaching them how to ski at Lake Tahoe. We would live near the vineyards and eat fresh California vegetables and drink lots of wine. I could see it all and it looked perfect, but for now the only real decision that needed to be made was which bar to hit with our friends and the only looming question was whether or not tomorrow would be a powder day.

I touched the wine label that was almost dry from the heat of the candle. Clos Du Bois, Alexander Valley, Chardonnay, 1984. It looked pretty on the white tablecloth. I reached into my bag and took out a glue stick and my journal and quickly glued the label onto a blank page. The pages of the book were filling quickly with the memories of Tony that I wanted to hold on to: ticket stubs from concerts we had been to, dried petals from the flowers he had given me, and other labels from bottles of wine we had drunk together.

A popping cork snapped my mind away from Boulder and back to the restaurant in St. Michaels. The waitress poured the wine. She carefully laid the bottle in the ice bucket and walked away from the table. I looked into Tony's eyes and it was like looking into a mirror. They were empty, tired and sad. I was sinking back into my life without Josie. I could tell he was already there.

They say that grief comes in waves. We had enjoyed a few hours together but now our time was up and the wave was knocking us down. We struggled through the dinner like a young couple on a bad date. We tried to talk about work, the weather, the children, the future, anything, but what lay between us was too massive. I wanted to reach out to him. I could feel his pain, see him struggling, but I couldn't help him because I couldn't help myself. Josie was dead, our lives were in ruin, and we could not bear to talk about it for fear of bringing the other one down even deeper.

The food came and we ate and drank because that was the only thing we could do. But the food had no taste. And the wine . . . I began thinking that perhaps being an alcoholic would not be such a bad thing. Alcoholics drank because the alcohol made the pain go away, and frankly, what was wrong with that? We had problems. We had pain. So why not drink and let it all go away?

As I gulped down my fourth glass of wine, I came to the realization that being here, alone together, was not a good thing, at least not now. We needed to be at home with the children, wiping up spilled milk, calling out spelling words, and making lunches. We needed to be with them. We needed distraction and constant motion.

We skipped dessert and left the restaurant. We didn't say much as we walked back to the hotel, and what little we did say felt forced and awkward. We were both lost in our own thoughts and pain.

I lay in bed that night next to Tony, realizing that perhaps our being together was toxic. I knew that many married couples who lose a child end up in divorce. As I lay there, I wondered what it would be like to be with another man, a man who was not weak like me, a man who was not grieving the loss of his beloved daughter, a man who had nothing else to worry about but me.

I turned to Tony as the tears slid down my face.

"Can we go home in the morning?"

"We'll go first thing." He wrapped his arm around me and I closed my eyes.

I woke up the next morning and Tony was gone. My head was pounding as I ran to the toilet to throw up. I swallowed some aspirin and wondered if Tony had been thinking the same thing I was last night. I imagined him with a beautiful woman who was happy and strong and would take care of him each day and nurse him back to life. Maybe he had taken an early morning bus to somewhere far away from me. I wouldn't blame him if he did. I put a wet washcloth on my forehead, crawled back under the sheets, and closed my eyes.

I heard the door open and Tony walked in with two cups of coffee.

"It's beautiful out. Let's do this ride. The guy at the coffee shop said it's really pretty. Come on, it'll make you feel better."

"I can't. I just threw up and my head is throbbing."

"That's all right, you'll be fine. Just drink the coffee. I got you a bagel and cream cheese. Get dressed. I'll get the bikes."

I sat on the curb and watched Tony as he pumped air into the tire of the yellow Greg LeMond that he had given me for my birthday. I thought about the last time I had sat on the bike. It was in the late fall. Josie had been fourteen months old.

I climbed on the bike and started pedaling, concentrating on following his blue shirt. I tucked myself behind his rear wheel, drafting, letting him cut through the stiff wind. The town, the pine trees, the farms with their families and their lives flew past us as the sun blazed down on our backs.

My mind tried to push me over into that dark pit of anger and sadness but I found that the harder and faster I moved my legs, the more I was able to stand at the pit and look down into it without being afraid. Tony picked up the pace and I pushed to keep up. I was in the hospital again. I was asking for help. No one was listening. Josie was dying in my arms. I was screaming inside and it was all coming out on the bike as the miles flew by.

I grabbed an energy bar and took a few bites. I rode up next to Tony. Handing him the other half, I pushed my bike in front of his. The tears and sweat dripped down my face and I wiped them away and pushed as fast as I could go. Somewhere. Anywhere.

We crossed the little metal bridge onto Tilghman Island. We didn't stop to take in the 360-degree view of the bay. We didn't stop to watch the local fire department as it prepared for a crab and corn feast. We circled around the island and headed back over the bridge with the wind at our backs. Tony pushed in front of me and I let his rear tire pull away from me as I gave my legs a rest. He sped away, his blue shirt getting smaller and smaller. I was sure he was thinking of Josie, too. The sadness was making me tired and I felt drained like I always did after a long session of grief therapy.

I saw Tony stop in the distance and as I began to gain on him, I could see him hunched over his bike.

"I've got a flat. Do you have an extra tube?" he asked.

Of course I didn't. I always relied on him for that kind of stuff.

"Do you want to ride on back to the hotel, and I'll walk and see if anyone can give me a lift," he asked as he wiped the grease off his hands.

"No, let's just walk back together."

I didn't want him to be alone, and I didn't want to be alone. I got off my bike and we walked side by side back to St. Michaels. The cars sped past us.

The clumping of our bike shoes broke the silence.

"Are we going to be all right?" I asked. "How are we going to survive this?"

"It's gonna be okay. We've just got to keep looking forward," he said. "We've gotta keep moving ahead."

We arrived home and it was good to see the children. They had had twenty-four fun-filled hours of movies, junk food, and a visit to the toy store. Twenty-four hours of not having to watch their parents struggle. Twenty-four hours of being spoiled rotten by their cheery aunt and grandmother, and they deserved every minute of it.

I had begun talking to a grief therapist and at one of the sessions she asked me how the trip had gone. I told her it was horrible. It had been a disaster because it was too hard to be alone together. "Maybe we're just no good for each other anymore," I said. "It's too painful for both of us."

"Sorrel, this is exactly why grieving parents get divorced. You are both sinking and you can't help each other buckle your life jackets. Think about Josie. Do you think she would want this? Do you think she would want Jack, Relly, and Eva to have to deal with a divorce on top of all that *they're* going through? Do you think that getting a divorce will make the pain go away? Grief is work: hard, hard work and you can *never* run away from it. It will always be with you. But you need to stop thinking about yourself."

9

Paul Bekman, our lawyer, was busy at work preparing our case against Johns Hopkins. I was still skeptical about Paul but I was eager to move the case forward. I fantasized about taking the stand.

"Mrs. King, you testified that you repeatedly raised concerns about Josie's dehydration to the medical staff. You testified that you asked for additional doctors and nurses to examine her. You testified that you asked that the 1:00 p.m. dose of methadone be withheld, and that a verbal order to withhold the methadone was given by the doctor. Is that true?"

"Yes. That is true."

"What happened at 1:00 p.m.?"

"The nurse came over with a syringe of methadone. I told her not to give it to Josie. I told her that there had been orders for no methadone to be given."

"What happened next, Mrs. King?"

"She squirted the methadone into Josie's mouth."

"And then what?"

"She had a cardiac arrest."

I knew the jury would eat this up. I knew the media would eat this up. I wanted the world to see how stupid and senseless her death had been. I wanted to see Hopkins suffer.

But there would be no media circus. There would be no destruction. There would be only one meeting, held six months after Josie died, in a conference room at Hopkins. On one side of the large table sat the Hopkins team, including Dr. George Dover and, of course, Rick Kidwell. Tony and I sat on the opposite side of the table with Paul Bekman.

The head of nursing began to nervously read through the results of the root cause analysis investigation. As I listened to her read on, thumbing through her piles of paper, reiterating everything we already knew, I wondered what the point of all of this was. We knew exactly what had happened, and so did they. I raised my hand.

"Does it say in your report that Josie's weight dropped dramatically in twenty-four hours?" I asked.

"Yes, it does."

"It was the residents' job to notice that, wasn't it?"

"Yes, it was."

"Why didn't they do something?"

There was no answer.

Rick Kidwell interrupted, "They should have noticed, but they didn't."

"May I ask you another question?"

"Go ahead," Rick replied.

"Why didn't the nurse call the doctor on Tuesday night when I saw that something was wrong?"

"They really thought she was fine. Her vitals were stable and that was what they were looking at."

"Do you think that Josie would be alive if she had been seen by a doctor that night?"

"I really can't answer with certainty, but I suspect so."

Tony interjected, "What I don't understand is why Josie was given a dose of the methadone when there had been an order that none be given."

"After examining Josie, the pain management team decided that she should be given the methadone," Rick explained.

I was dumbfounded. I could not understand what the team saw in Josie that morning that could possibly have made them think the methadone was needed.

The nurse explained that when a patient has been on methadone, the weaning must be carefully planned and monitored to avoid serious complications of withdrawal such as diarrhea and an upset stomach. These symptoms can lead to more serious complications such as convulsions and neurological damage. The team did not want this to happen to Josie, especially since she had shown flu-like symptoms a few days earlier.

"Are you suggesting that the methadone had nothing to do with her going into cardiac arrest?" I asked.

"Yes, that is what we believe," Rick said.

"Tell me then, what did she die of?" I demanded.

There was silence as the tension in the room rose. Tony and I looked at each other. He leaned back in his chair and crossed his arms over his chest. Paul Bekman put his pen down and laid his hands on the table. The three of us looked at Rick and waited for an answer.

"Well," Rick paused, "there were complications."

I pounced back. "Rick, she died because she was dehydrated and was then given a narcotic. It was the combination of the two. It was because you all didn't listen and pay attention, and you know it!"

"Mrs. King, she should not have died," he said. "And yes, you're right. She would probably be alive if we had listened."

The anger was boiling up inside me, overtaking my sadness, creating a powerful energy that made me feel as if it would send me rocketing through the glass window if I stood up. I gripped the armrests of the chair.

They had said what I wanted to hear, but it wasn't enough.

A few weeks later, Paul came to our house and handed us the legal documents from Hopkins. There it was: the settlement offer. It was a concept that was difficult to comprehend— money for the death of our daughter. The thought of us accepting it was almost as appalling as them offering it. We didn't want their money and felt that by accepting it we would be letting them off the hook. We didn't want it to be so easy for them.

Tony told Paul that we'd have to think about it.

In the days and weeks after Hopkins offered us the settlement I hit rock bottom. Family and friends were back in their routines and Tony was keeping his mind off things by staying busy at work. Jack, Relly, and Eva were in full swing at school. And I sat at home without Josie.

I began thinking horrible thoughts. I wanted to drive my car the hour and a half to Bruce Farm, turn on the cozy electric blanket, and swallow the contents of a king-size bottle of aspirin. I wanted to close my eyes and drift off to sleep to be with Josie.

Dr. Watson was the first of many grief therapists. I had chosen her because she, too, had lost a child. I figured she would be a good person to talk to, that she could sympathize. I sat in her office and talked about my sadness and anger, looking at the photo of her child propped on her desk.

One day, I decided I would tell her what I was really thinking. "Sometimes I think about what it would be like to just end it all." I waited for her reaction, for her to call the hotline for the really seriously screwed-up people, for her to run over to the sofa and beg me not to pull the trigger, but she didn't.

She told me that when her child had died she had also had these kinds of thoughts. "There are books and Web sites on how to do it," she said.

She might as well have handed me the how-to manual. I struggled through the rest of the session feeling as if I were being led down a path I now no longer wanted to be on. She closed her notebook to signal that we were done.

I sat in my car and thought about the bizarre conversation that had just occurred. Either she was an excellent therapist and had just pulled some good reverse psychology or she was sick and tired of my whining and no longer wanted me around. One thing she had made clear to me was that my feelings for wanting to end my life were natural and that if I really wanted to I could find a way to go through with it. This reality frightened me. It made me realize that I didn't really want to leave. I had to stay.

Jack turned seven and I could barely arrange a birthday party. We all stood around the dining room table as he blew out the candles on the Spider-Man cake that I had bought at the grocery store. I pulled up a chair and sat next to him as I felt that familiar sensation of tears beginning to form. Josie would have liked to be here. *She would have wanted to put her chubby little fingers in the cake, she would have wanted to blow out the candles, and she would have wanted to rip open Jack's presents,* I thought as the tears slid down my face.

"What did you wish for?" Relly asked.

I cringed, not wanting to have to explain to Jack that his wish for Josie to come home would never come true. I looked at Tony.

"If you tell your wish it will never come true," Tony said.

Jack looked at me and then at Tony. "I wish Mom would stop crying," he said as he stuck the knife into the cake.

His words struck me like a bolt of lightning and I realized that my children had not only lost their little sister but they were slowly losing their mother. I was letting it happen before their very eyes. My pain and my sadness, the ungodly sight of it, was causing them further anguish. I wiped my tears away not knowing what to say. I passed the Spider-Man plates around the table. "Sometimes my eyes just water because of my contact lenses," I said, knowing he could see right through me.

I would sit alone in Josie's room. I could hear Gloria downstairs answering the phone, washing dishes, handling everything. She was from Trinidad and at fifty years old she had not a wrinkle on her round silky face, which was framed by a shoulder-length 1970s feathered haircut. We had hired her to help us get settled when we moved to Baltimore. Originally a part-time helper, she had now become a full-fledged member of the family. Every now and then Gloria would come into Josie's room to check on me.

"Come on, girl. It's time for you to get up and come downstairs. You need to pick out the tile for the countertop."

"You can pick it out, Gloria. Just pick something black."

She told me it was time to get out of that room. "You come on down and look at them. It's time for lunch," she said. "We can have some soup together."

I followed her downstairs. She and Wes, the builder, showed me the tiles. I looked at all the shades of black, some shiny, some matte.

"I don't know, Gloria, what do you think?" I asked.

She pointed to a black-honed granite. "That one is pretty."

"Okay," I said, as I started back up the steps.

"You can't spend all day in that room," she said sternly. "Come back here and eat some lunch."

We sat at the table together as we had done so many times before with Josie in her high chair between us. Sometimes, on warm sunny days, Gloria and I had taken our lunch outside to the terrace, where she would sit in the shade of the magnolia tree and I would stay in the sun with Josie. Now we sat at the table with the empty high chair between us.

"I think we need to get rid of the chair. This afternoon I'm going to put it in the garage. It's time for you to get used to not seeing it," she said, eating a spoonful of her tomato soup.

"Okay," I said, letting the tears trickle down my face.

"We gotta keep on movin' down the road."

"I know," I said. "I just miss her."

"I bought you something." She handed me a package wrapped in white tissue paper. I opened it and held up a blue sundress with pink flowers. "I think it's time for you to get out of this house. You need to fix yourself up. You and Tony need to go out to dinner and go dancing."

It had been months since I had left the house to do anything other than what was absolutely necessary—taking the children to and from school and sports practices, and getting groceries. The thought of putting on a dress and doing something fun seemed foreign to me. I wanted to stay in the house with Gloria and my family and hide from the world just a little bit longer.

Gloria took over. Every time she relayed a question to me from the architect, the builder, or the electrician, I told her I didn't care and that they could decide without me. She became the consultant to them all. She was the boss of the house, the decision maker, my psychotherapist, my babysitter, and my friend.

I was coming to the realization that our story was like an urban legend, except it was the real thing. Friends would tell me that strangers on the chair lift in Vermont had been talking about "that poor family in Baltimore."

My mother came up from Richmond to take Relly and Eva out to buy Easter dresses. She knew I wouldn't do it myself. We went to the Pied Piper, a children's store down the road. I wanted to be back at home where I felt safe, where I didn't have to pretend I was normal. My mother and the girls looked at dresses as I stood by wishing that we were buying three dresses instead of two.

I noticed a young mother over by the sweater display looking at me and whispering to the saleslady. She caught my eye, quickly looked away, and ran out the door leaving her shopping bags behind. I walked over to my mother and the saleslady and asked them what had happened.

The saleslady looked at me and then at my mother.

"I guess she recognized you and was just so sad she had to leave," my mother said as she put her arm around my shoulder and led me over to the hair bands.

I looked out the window, wondering if the woman would come back for her bags. How dare she cry? She had nothing to cry about. Didn't she know how lucky she was? Didn't she know that I was using every ounce of my energy to be standing in this stupid store?

We live in a country where to most people death is an uncommon thing. Mothers rarely die during childbirth anymore. We have created powerful vaccines to keep our children from dying of typhoid fever, malaria, or cholera. It is uncommon for Americans to freeze to death in the winter or die of starvation. I remember thinking that perhaps I should have been living in those earlier times—the frontier days—when death was a common occurrence. I pictured myself with the other mothers who had lost their children to various ailments. We would churn butter all day and go about our grieving together. Then I realized that it would not have mattered what era I lived in. No matter how many other mothers I was with, my heart would still be broken, and Josie would still be gone.

The grief books say that your friends change when someone you love dies. Sometimes the person who you were good friends with, who you thought would be there for you, chooses to run away from you and your misery. And sometimes a complete stranger will help you in ways you never thought possible. As a grieving mother, I was quickly beginning to figure out who and what worked for me.

One afternoon a few weeks after Josie died, the doorbell rang. It was my friend Elizabeth with her eighteen-month-old daughter, Katy. She told me she was on her way to take Katy to music class but was running early.

"I just wanted to see how you were doing," she said, balancing Katy on her hip.

As they walked in the door I looked past her and noticed that the crocuses and daffodils were just beginning to pop out of the ground. I slowly began realizing that life for everyone else was moving on and that the earth, too, had decided it would not stop revolving just because Josie had died. Winter was turning into spring.

I quickly shut the door behind them. The last eighteen-month-old I had seen was Josie. Katy, oblivious to the pain she was causing me, waddled over to the snack cabinet and reached up.

"Oh, can she have one of those juice boxes?" Elizabeth asked.

I felt like I was moving in slow motion, reliving something that I had done so many times before for Josie. I reached up for the little green box and took the straw off, ripped the plastic away, and poked it into the little silver hole, being careful not to squeeze it. My hands trembled. I concentrated on holding back the tears as I handed the box to Katy, feeling as if I were betraying Josie. She grabbed it from my hand and ran to her mother, away from me and the look in my eyes.

I did my best to listen to Elizabeth as she asked me how I was. I told her I was fine as I watched Katy play with one of Josie's dolls, but I wanted to rip it out of her hands. I stumbled through the awkward conversation and finally told her I had a headache and that maybe we could visit another day. They left. I didn't want to see my friend or her daughter. I didn't want to see the flowers blooming or winter turning into spring. I shut the door on the world that should have stopped when Josie died.

I sat on the steps and put my hand on the spot where, just a few weeks earlier, I had sat with Josie as she drank her juice box and I had sipped my coffee. She always squeezed the box too tightly, letting the juice dribble over. I would lean over and wipe it up, never realizing how lucky I was.

Friends occasionally caused me pain, but sometimes complete strangers or people I barely knew would rise out of nowhere and provide me with strength and comfort. Wes, the builder, was a big strong man with graying hair and a mustache. He wore jeans and a tool belt and he and his two-man crew, Joe and Dave, had been working on the old green-shingle farmhouse for a few months. Every morning that they came to work I'd have a pot of coffee waiting for them. While Jack, Relly, and Eva were at school Josie had watched them pour concrete, saw the sheets of plywood, and hammer in the nails. She smiled when they handed her a tape measure or a wax pencil to play with.

And then one day they came to work and it was all gone. The cute little girl who squealed when they picked her up was dead and her mother was no longer the person they once knew. They didn't play their loud AC/DC on the boom box anymore, and they didn't scream at each other from across the house. I could hear them quietly working and talking in hushed voices while Gloria made them coffee. Sometimes, when Gloria made me come downstairs, they'd peek in at me sitting at the kitchen table with her. Gloria would motion for them to come over and join us at the table and they sat and talked while I listened.

Wes told me about his mother who had died long ago and how she had made the best homemade macaroni and cheese.

"I know they're up there in heaven together. Don't worry," he said. "Josie's all right. My mother is taking good care of her."

I asked him if he believed in heaven. "Darn right I do," he said. "And I bet they're up there right now eating macaroni and cheese."

Joe and Dave nodded in agreement. If only I knew there was a heaven. If only I knew she was all right. I asked them to turn their music back up and not to feel like they had to tiptoe around me. "Just be like you were," I said.

As the days and weeks passed they'd see me and just shake their heads. One day Gloria brought Joe and Dave into Josie's room where I was sitting. She told me it was time. I watched as they dismantled the crib. They carried it out piece by piece and put it in the barn, leaving only a bag of screws on the bureau. "Let's paint this room a pretty color and let Eva sleep in it," she suggested.

They didn't know it at the time, but Wes, Joe, and Dave helped me through the dark days. These three big strong men, whom I barely knew, took care of me as if they were my oldest friends. Their music, their voices, the progress happening beneath my feet gave me something else to think about, something else to listen to other than the silence.

10

As the months wore on I would rarely pick up the phone, so people would leave messages. "Checking in," they would say, or "Thinking of you." "Let me know what I can do." Sometimes a stranger would leave a message. A mother would explain that she had also lost her child and she knew what I was going through. She would always leave a number for me to call when I was ready.

When the children were asleep, I would sneak down and call these strangers. It helped to know that there were others like me, and that they had survived. The mothers were anywhere between two and sixteen years into their grief, and I had become part of their sisterhood.

Alice had had a six-year-old son named James. Her husband was driving a motor boat when James fell off the back, got sucked under the boat, and died. When I talked to Alice, she was five years into her grief. Karen's five-year-old son, Ethan, died from leukemia, two years before Josie. Gina lived a few miles down the road from me; her sixteen-year-old daughter, Casey, had died in a horseback-riding accident while at camp.

The mother I talked to the most was from the west coast. Her name was Rachel. She had thought she had found the perfect nanny for her three-year-old, named Lucas. What she did not know was that the nanny had a gambling addiction, and on a hot August day the nanny drove Lucas with her to the slot machines. She left him locked in the car for five hours while she fed her addiction. Lucas died of severe dehydration and heat stroke.

When I first began talking to Rachel, she was three years into her grief. We spoke every few weeks. I asked if she was happy and she said she was. She told me she was profoundly happy. "One day you will be happy, too." I did not want to hear these words. How could she be happy without her son and how could she possibly think that I could ever be happy without Josie? The thought actually made me sick to my stomach. Yet I tucked her words deep in my brain.

Rachel talked a lot about religion and how God had helped her through it all. One day she told me she was studying to become a minister. She told me that she was going out to the state prison to share Holy Communion with the nanny who had been sentenced to ten years for killing her son. She was going to forgive her.

"Sorrel, are you there?" she asked as I sat in shock three thousand miles away.

The only words I could think of were, "Are you out of your mind?"

I didn't talk to Rachel again for a long time. I just couldn't understand where she was coming from. I felt as if she were betraying her son.

Like Rachel, every single one of the other women I talked to said that she had found comfort in God and religion. Their words kept ringing in my head.

"God showed me the way."

"My church was just wonderful."

"My faith really helped me."

"I could not have survived without my parish."

"Let God help you."

These women had something I did not and I often felt embarrassed and ashamed to admit that I didn't really believe in God. I told them I wished I could see things the way they did. The more I talked to them, the more I realized that I needed to find God. If religion helped them, surely it would help me. I just needed to figure out how.

Church was a place we had been forced to go to as children and I had hated it. I hated having to wake up on a beautiful Sunday morning, put on nice clothes, drive downtown, and sit still for an hour and a half. The worst part was Sunday school. I was friends with Annie Gray, the preacher's daughter, and the two of us would sometimes sneak out of Sunday school, walk down Broad Street, and get some fries and a shake at the McDonald's nearby. We used the money from our Unicef boxes, telling ourselves that we would put our next week's allowance in the box.

If we were not at McDonald's, Annie would sneak us into her father's office. It was a big beautiful room with a window that looked out onto a pretty garden. He had a huge desk with leather chairs and a green leather sofa. The walls were covered with books on religion, psychology, science, death, and poetry. Sometimes we heard footsteps and dove behind the sofa. There was always a big sigh of relief when the intruder was just another one of our friends sneaking out of Sunday school class.

When church was over it would take twenty-five minutes to pull my mother away from her various conversations. What was the point of it all? Couldn't we achieve the same thing by reading a poem, saying a prayer, or singing a hymn while we were walking in the woods? Isn't nature God's house, and wouldn't He rather have us enjoying what He created. And what was with the getting dressed up? Does God really care what we wear? Every Sunday I asked my parents these questions. I don't remember their responses but I know I was never convinced.

As I grew into a teenager, a college student, a single girl living in New York City, and then a wife and mother, my feelings for church and religion never changed. I just didn't get it. Even though I was unsure about God and religion I *was* sure of one thing—I believed there was someone or something much more powerful than ourselves, and that there was a plan for each of us, a purpose.

I began my search for religion at the Ivy Book Shop, a little bookstore down the road from us in Baltimore. I walked up and down the self-help and religion aisles and picked up whatever books looked simple and straightforward. I started with Deepak Chopra's *How to Know God*. I also tuned my car radio to the religious stations. I hoped that perhaps, if I drove around in my car listening to religious music, maybe I would find help through osmosis. I also decided that meeting with a minister would help clear things up.

The minister I called was from a local church. He looked young, perhaps in his mid-thirties. I was skeptical. We sat in his office and he listened as I told him my story. Tears streamed down my face, my nose ran, and the sleeve of my sweater got wet and soggy from wiping it all up. He sat, looked, and listened from across the room. He asked if I had forgiven Hopkins, said that perhaps it would make me feel better if I did. He explained to me how God had forgiven the people who had crucified his very own son, Jesus.

Forgiveness. It was a concept I could not comprehend. I sat in disbelief as he rambled on about forgiveness. How could I believe in a God that wanted me to forgive the people who had killed my daughter?

"I don't understand what you're saying," I said as I wiped away my tears. "I can't see things the way you do." I stood up and told him that I planned on doing everything I could to destroy Hopkins, then walked out of the room.

Where was the wise old white-haired minister who had lost a brother in the war or a wife to cancer? He would have handed me some tissues. He would have sat next to me and said, "I don't blame you for being angry."

In September of 2001, seven months after Josie died, our country was faced with the unspeakable tragedy of 9/11. I sat with the congregation that first Sunday after the terrorist attacks as we all waited for the minister to walk down the aisle, stand behind the pulpit, and share with us words that would help us understand

Three thousand people died that day. Wives lost husbands and husbands lost wives; children lost parents and parents lost children. Added to that grief was our country's lost sense of security and comfort. It was all over the media: death, destruction, and disbelief. As each day passed, emotions reeled and people tried desperately to make sense of it all.

Radio station talk shows and television news programs scrambled to deliver information on topics such as grief, depression, and post-traumatic stress disorder. I was no longer alone in mourning.

The minister proceeded to talk, not about the victims or their families, but about the terrorists. He explained to the congregation that the terrorists were God's children and that God loved them as well as us. Once again, I could not believe what I was hearing. How could he possibly be saying this? Would he be using such words if it had been his child that had been forced to jump out of a window a hundred stories up, or if it had been his wife who was in the plane that crashed into the building, or if his brother had been a fireman climbing up fifty flights of stairs to rescue people when tons of concrete and metal collapsed on him? How could he? I looked around, thinking that maybe I was missing something. Maybe I was overly sensitive. People whispered into their neighbors' ears. They shook their heads.

I joined a church group, figuring that being with a group of women who spent an hour or two out of the week "nourishing their souls" might be a good place for me, and I gravitated to the older members of the group. I felt I had more in common with the seventy- to eighty-year-old set than the members who were my age. These older women were kind and sensitive. They knew my story and why I was there.

We sat in a circle on metal folding chairs and at the beginning of each session we held hands and sang a song. This was when, as hard as I tried not to, my tears would start flowing. I would let go of the hands and leave the room, searching for an empty classroom where I could bury my head. After the third week or so of this, the leader told me it was okay to cry, that I should not leave the room. I nodded my head and remained in place, crying, as the ladies held hands and sang. After the singing we would break into small discussion groups. Most of the time I just listened and hoped that today would be the day that something would click, that I would discover God.

One day, in the small group session, one of the women began to cry. I looked at her, wondering if she and I shared something in common. Perhaps she had suffered a loss, too. Maybe there was someone who could share my lonely world. She told the group between sobs that her horse had died. The women all rose to comfort her. I sat, paralyzed.

That was my last day with the group. I realized then that I was in the wrong place. I didn't belong there. I told myself that even if I did find God, Josie would still be gone. My grief was overwhelming. I needed professional help.

I was no longer seeing Dr. Watson and Josie's pediatrician, Dr. Bogue, recommended Sandra Fink. Sandra was a grief therapist who worked for a local hospice. She had had her fair share of patients who were dying from terminal illnesses, parents who had lost children, children who had lost parents, and much more. Dealing with death was her thing.

Her office was in a hospice center's basement at the end of a long, dark hall lit up by a Coke machine, and there was a white plastic chair next to the door. As I plopped myself down on the chair to wait, the tears began to fall. The janitor was sweeping the floor and looked at me. I am sure he was used to seeing pathetic people like me sitting outside this office crying, waiting for some magical cure.

The door opened and I wiped away the tears as the previous visitor quietly left the room. She glanced at me and I wondered, as I watched her disappear down the dark hall, what her story was. I knew that, like me, she had some serious problems. Was she dying of breast cancer? Had her husband just died? Had she, too, lost a child? Whatever it was, we had something in common.

I liked Sandra the minute I saw her. She wore a pretty, flower-print pastel dress that matched her pale pink lipstick and she had a tan complexion and grayish, blonde hair with bangs. She invited me in. "Ahh, Sorrel," she said as she put her arms around me.

We sat down. Her windowless office had rattan furniture that was painted white and a big glass coffee table with a bowl of sea glass and pretty garden books on it. The pictures that hung on the walls were of beach scenes with glass panes, giving one the failed illusion that you were at a beach house with a water view.

She asked me to tell her my story, Josie's story. Every time I stopped to control my sobs, she waited patiently, handed me another tissue, and then told me to go on. I kept going over the events at the hospital, as if the more I talked about it, the greater the chance was that Josie would not have died. Every session began like this and at the end of each session I was exhausted and tired of crying.

Sometimes I would come in and ask if she could prescribe medication that would make the pain go away. She told me there were drugs that could maybe help in the short term, but down the road things would only be worse. There was no such thing as a quick fix to grief.

"Grieving," she said, "is hard, hard work. You can't go under it. You can't go around it. You can only go through it." She told me that there was no road map or manual to make it any easier, but she did have a suggestion for me. "Try something new," she said. "This will force your mind to focus on something else and will give you breaks from the grief."

Starting something new was a concept I could grasp. This was concrete advice and I could do it. I left her office that day with a plan. I called my friend Laura, who had given birth to a stillborn child six months before Josie died, and I told her what Sandra had suggested. We met at the music store that afternoon and she left with a fiddle and I with an acoustic Fender guitar.

I found a teacher who came to the house and gave me guitar lessons. I also bought a sketchbook and some pastels and made the children pose for me as I drew their faces. The thing I liked most, though, was sanding the unfinished furniture that I had bought. While the children were at school I would spend hours sanding the two beds and the bureau I had set up in the driveway. I sanded the pieces using every muscle in my body. The anger came through my hands as I moved the sandpaper faster and harder across the pine. I could not stop until the muscles in my back and arms screamed. I kept going until my fingers bled. The harder and longer I sanded, the more pain I felt, but the physical pain felt good. It allowed me to focus on something other than the emptiness I felt in my heart.

Jack, Relly, and Eva arrived home from school to see their mother bent over, sanding furiously with bloody hands while sweat and tears streamed down her face. I asked them how school was. They told me it was fine. They looked at the pile of discarded sandpaper strewn across the driveway.

"Are you doing this because you miss Josie?" Relly asked.

Sandra had told me that it was okay to let the children see me grieve for Josie but that they needed to also see me as the happy mother I had once been. I handed them each a piece of sandpaper. "Sure I miss Josie, but this is fun," I said. "It's easy. Try it."

And so we all sanded in the afternoon and they told me about their day. Josie was not on their mind constantly the way she was on mine and I was grateful for that. The two red-stained beds, made from blood, sweat, and tears, are still in Jack's room.

Writing had always been a way for me to get the swirling thoughts out of my brain, and after Josie died I continued to put pen to paper. It helped me work through problems. Two days after her death, I bought a journal and sat in her room and wrote all day. Like the journal I kept in the hospital, my days were no longer Monday, Tuesday, and Wednesday. They were numbered, day one, day two, day three: a count of the days gone by without Josie.

Day 10. Today I looked across the lawn and imagined you running to me. I picked you up and swung you around. You are gone. I will never touch you again. I will never see you again. I will never hear your sweet little voice say "night, night" or "mine, mine, mine." Why did you have to go? Why did this have to happen? Josie, you were so brave . . .

When I wasn't writing in my notebook, I was pounding furiously on the computer keyboard late at night, after the children had gone to sleep. Writing felt good. I could write evil, horrible things, and no one could hear me. It felt productive.

Books were another thing that helped me. I bought every book I could find on losing a child. Just as I liked talking to grieving mothers, I could read endlessly about people who had gone through what I was going through: the father whose wife, daughter, and mother were killed by a drunk driver; the mother whose two daughters died in a car accident; the father whose son died in a climbing accident. I could relate to the people in these books. They became my friends and every night I would get in bed and, for a little while, escape with them into their sad world and feel their pain. Not only did the books give me people whom I could relate to, they also gave me hope that somehow, like them, I, too, would survive.

11

Paul Bekman, our lawyer, was beginning to worry. It had been weeks since Hopkins had made their offer and we still had not accepted the settlement. The notion of us not taking the money was beginning to look like a reality.

Paul came to the house one evening in August. We went into the living room and sat down and he told us we needed to make a decision on the settlement offer. "Hopkins is not going to let this stand indefinitely," he said.

"Josie's worth more than that," I replied.

"You're not going to get more." He had explained this to me over and over again. Maryland has a settlement cap of a little less than 1.5 million dollars for this type of situation, which includes pain and suffering—my and Tony's pain and suffering, and Josie's pain and suffering. If it had been Tony who had died, the settlement would have been considerably more because Tony has economic value—lost wages to account for. In the eyes of Maryland law, Josie—a minor— was of lesser economic value.

There it was, my primer on the world of malpractice caps and tort reform. Every time Paul explained it to me I told him it didn't make sense; it wasn't fair. And every time he told me the same thing.

"That's how the legal system works."

"We don't care what they offer us. We still don't want to sign the papers," I said.

Tony explained to him that this seemed like just a drop in the bucket for Hopkins, a small slap on the wrist. "If we take this money, we'll be letting them off the hook. It seems too easy for them."

"Let's just take it to a jury and see what happens," I said. "You know we'll win, and you know the media will be all over it. Let's see what Hopkins does then."

"If we go to court it could take years," he answered. "It will be grueling, not only for the two of you, but also for your children. You want to destroy Hopkins? Well, Hopkins will do the same to you. There is no doubt in my mind that we would win, *but* you will only walk away with what has already been offered in this settlement. You gain nothing by going to court."

"I want everyone to know what they did. If we don't go to court, the media won't pick up on it. Hopkins is only going to hide it and forget that it ever happened," I said.

"We can call the media right now and there could be a story in tomorrow's paper, but you know what? It will be one sad story in one local paper and then it will be forgotten."

I told him it was all wrong. None of what he was saying was making it any easier to take the money. "We don't want their money," I reiterated.

"What *do* you want?" he asked.

I told him that I wanted them to remember Josie, to learn something from her and to never let this happen again. "I want every hospital in the country to know her name and why she died. I want them *all* to learn something," I said angrily.

"Then do that," he said. "Do that with the settlement money. If you leave this money, it will just get sucked up in a black hole." He paused and picked up the settlement papers. "Take the money and do something good. Do something for Josie. You can make this more than a sad story for the media to cover. You can create something much more."

I thought about it. As much as I wanted a fight in court, maybe he was right. It could take years and it could be painful. It would just be a sensationalized courtroom battle story, and for what? I looked at Tony.

"I think he's right," he said. "I think we should take the money and do something good with it."

And so we took the money. We signed the papers, and a few days later Paul handed us a check.

I walked into our local bank on Roland Avenue, a place that I had often visited, usually with Josie on my hip and a cup of Stone Mill coffee in my hand. I held the check in my hand as I stood in line.

"Welcome to Wachovia. How are you today, Mrs. King?" Christy the teller asked as I approached her window.

I endorsed the check and slid it over. I watched her look at the check, waiting for her to notice that this was not my normal Friday transaction. I wanted to tell her where the money had come from and how hard it was for me to be doing what I was doing. I wanted this moment to mean something. I watched her, waiting for her to say something, but she looked up at me and asked the same old question.

"Would you like any cash back, Mrs. King?"

12

One day, not long after we accepted the settlement, Sandra said something to me that transformed the way that I grieved for Josie.

"This energy from your grief and anger is very powerful. It's time for you to make a decision," she told me. "You can let the grief and anger continue to destroy you. You can sit in your house all day, cry, and be angry at Hopkins and the world. You can give up. Or you can take that energy and use it to propel yourself forward." She took a sip of her tea and looked at me. "Get out there and *do* something with your anger. *Do* something with your pain."

I thought back to my childhood, to happier times and summers at Bruce Farm in Virginia, when my mother—wearing blue jeans, a bathing-suit top, and holding a riding crop—would stand in the middle of the lawn and give us riding lessons. "Heads up and heels down," she'd command as we jumped over cross rails, galloped through fields, and sailed over stone walls. When one of us got bucked off she'd pick us up, wipe our tears away, check our bodies for broken bones, and then make us get back in the saddle. "If you fall off a horse, you get right back on," she'd say as we pleaded to quit.

I came home that day thinking about what Sandra had said. I thought back to when the neurologists told me Josie was going to die: how I realized at that moment, in a flash, that something tremendous was happening. I knew from the very beginning that there had to be a reason that Josie was taken from me. And now I knew that reason was not for me to sit in my house all day and feel sorry for myself.

Sandra was right. I had to make a choice. Maybe the pain and sadness could be made into a form other than tears, a form much more powerful and productive. It was time to stop looking for God and religion to rescue me. It was time to put away the paints and the guitar, hoping for the pain to go away. It was time to do something else, something for Josie. Maybe, like Jack wanted, I should stop crying and maybe, like Gloria had said, it was time to leave Josie's room and get out of the house.

Tony and I began discussing what we would do with the money. Should we donate it to kids with cancer? Should we fund a playroom in the new Hopkins Children's Center? We knew we wanted to do something with children and hospitals. So, while Tony spent his days at work, I sat at the computer looking for ideas about what to do with the money.

It had to be huge, nationwide—worldwide even, earth-shatteringly tremendous. As I thought of all our options, there was one question that lurked in the back of my mind and there was only one person who could answer it.

I picked up the phone and called Rick Kidwell.

He was shocked to hear my voice and proceeded to tell me that I should not be contacting him unless it was through our lawyer. I told him it was over. We had signed the papers.

115

He put me on hold for a minute.

I knew as I sat there waiting that he was calling Paul Bekman to make sure Mrs. King hadn't totally lost it.

When he came back to me it was as if I was talking to an entirely different person. He apologized for Josie's death. He apologized for any pain that the legal proceedings may have caused us. He told me he was sorry.

I was caught off guard by his apology and so I just asked him straight, "Josie's death was a fluke. It was a strike of lightning. Medical errors like that don't happen very often, do they?"

He told me that people die every day from medical errors. "It's happening in hospitals everywhere. It's reported to be one of the leading causes of death in our country," he said.

I was shocked.

"No one really talks about it," he told me. "Doctors and nurses are not publicizing the fact, the patients are either dead or in the middle of a nasty legal battle, and the families are just too grief-stricken to do anything about it."

I hung up the phone that day and began searching the Internet for more information. The more I read, the more I was beginning to realize the magnitude of the problem.

A 2000 report by the Institute of Medicine, called *To Err Is Human,* found that between forty-four thousand and ninety-eight thousand people a year die from medical errors, the equivalent of a jumbo jet crashing every day. Deaths from medical errors, it concluded, was one of our country's top killers, along with cancer, AIDS, diabetes, and heart disease. The Joint Commission—the nation's premier health care safety and quality accreditation organization—reported that over

70 percent of all sentinel events, unexpected medical events that result in death or serious injury, occur because of a breakdown in communication—just like what happened to Josie.

Every night when Tony came home from work, I told him everything I was learning about medical errors and patient safety.

We decided we'd start a foundation. Its mission would be to prevent patients from being harmed or killed by medical errors. We would name it after Josie, and we would begin with Johns Hopkins.

I knew that in order to make this work we needed someone within Hopkins who believed in what we wanted to do, someone we could trust with our blood money.

A good friend of ours, who happened to be a Hopkins doctor by the name of David Cromwell, called and told me he knew just the person to help us: Dr. Peter Pronovost, an anesthesiologist whose father had died from medical errors. Patient safety was his passion.

David told me that he had just attended a mandatory patient safety conference at which Dr. Pronovost had been speaking. He explained to me that these conferences are usually filled with dry statistics, lengthy PowerPoint presentations, and can often be downright boring. "This conference," he told me, "was different from any other. When Dr. Pronovost spoke, people closed their laptops and put their BlackBerries away. They listened to him. He not only moved the audience, he had people fired up."

I called Dr. Pronovost the next day. He said he would come to our house and meet with Tony and me. A few days later he stood in the doorway. What David neglected to tell me was that Peter looked like he was twenty-one. I told him I had thought he was much older when we had talked on the phone.

"I really don't feel like dealing with any more young doctors from Hopkins," I said, a bit sheepishly.

He promised me we were the same age. I let him in.

Peter was the lead researcher on quality and safety and had created a program called CUSP, the Comprehensive Unit-Based Safety Program. He talked at length about the program and his excitement was infectious. Patient safety was a culture thing, he said. It was about doctors and nurses listening to each other and listening to the patient or parent, it was about working out issues before they became incidents, it was about improving teamwork—it was about communication.

CUSP was a six-step program that addressed these very issues. The first step of the program was to measure the hospital culture. Peter did this by using a patient safety culture survey at the unit level, asking questions such as: Is teamwork on your unit effective? Is staffing an issue? Does management address your patient safety concerns? This survey provided Peter with a measurement of effectiveness, a baseline. "We need to know where we are so that we know where we're going," he said. The second step was to educate the caregivers on why safety is so important. Step number three was to identify issues. Peter would ask each unit the simple question, "How will the next patient be harmed?" The fourth step was to take those issues, prioritize them, and then use interdisciplinary teams to form projects to resolve them. Once those issues were resolved they became stories. Step number five was to share the stories—the lessons learned and the process changes that were made to improve safety and quality with other units and other hospitals. Finally, the last step was to resurvey the unit.

Peter's program made sense to us. As Tony and I listened it became apparent that if such a program had been in place at Hopkins, perhaps Josie would be alive today.

We liked Peter. He seemed passionate about what he did. He also told us about his family. He had a daughter named Emma who was the same age Josie would have been. As he looked at the picture of Josie that was lying on the coffee table, I could see his eyes fill with tears.

My Friday calls with George Dover continued but they were no longer filled with my threats. We now spoke about how Johns Hopkins and the Josie King Foundation were going to partner to prevent medical errors. We joined forces with Dr. Pronovost and six months later we gave a large portion of the settlement back to Hopkins. With the money, two CUSP programs were implemented on the floors where Josie had been cared for. The programs were to be called "The Josie King Pediatric Patient Safety Programs."

We were feeling good about these baby steps into the world of patient safety but I knew that this was just the beginning of the work we needed to do for Josie.

Rick Kidwell's words kept ringing in my head: *No one really talks about it.*

I wanted to talk about it. I wanted to stand before doctors and nurses and tell them Josie's story. I wanted every doctor and every nurse to know her name. I picked up the phone and called Rick. I told him I wanted to tell Josie's story.

"You should," he said. "People need to hear it. They'll listen to you."

I was surprised that he was giving me the go-ahead to air Hopkins' dirty laundry. In fact, he was encouraging me to do it. I wanted to share Josie's story because I wanted doctors and nurses to learn from the mistakes that Hopkins had made, but not all of my intentions were good. There was a part of me that wanted to share the story so that I could stick it to Hopkins. I didn't want it to be so easy for them.

A month later, Rick arranged for me to speak at Hopkins' grand rounds. Grand rounds, which are held in most academic hospitals, are typically hour-long sessions where information is shared, new procedures are taught, and new technology introduced. These meetings are conducted by doctors, nurses, or executives and are meant to be educational and informative for the hospital staff.

I stood behind the podium in wood-paneled Hurd Hall. The room was amphitheater-like and I looked up to the seats that rose above me, all the way to the balcony. There was standing room only, with a sea of white coats, scrubs, and business suits. I had never given a speech before, but today I was addressing some of the very people who had contributed to Josie's death. I had worked hard to craft my message. I so wanted to scream at them and tell them how much it hurt, but I knew if I told them how I really felt, they would leave the room, shake their heads, and say that Sorrel King had lost her mind. Besides, there were no words that could describe my pain.

Instead, I shared with them exactly what happened to Josie and how her care had fallen apart. I broke it down for them like a science experiment and kindly asked them to listen to each other, listen to the patients, and listen to the parents. I asked them to partner with me. I asked them to help me.

A few days later, Peter suggested that I travel with him to Boston to speak at an IHI conference. I was hesitant and told him that I didn't want to leave my children. I didn't even know what IHI stood for.

Peter explained to me that the IHI, the Institute for Healthcare Improvement, is an organization that works to improve quality and safety within our health care system. It had been cofounded in 1991 by Dr. Donald Berwick, a pediatrician from Boston, and a few other doctors who had seen the need to improve quality in American health care. They were witnessing too many errors occurring at the bedside. Other industries such as the airline industry, the nuclear power industry, and the automotive industry all focused on quality and safety but the health care industry had never before done so.

"They need to hear from you. They need to hear Josie's story," Peter said. "This is your chance to tell it to three hundred doctors, nurses, and administrators from around the country." He knew I couldn't say no because he knew how badly I wanted to get my story beyond the walls of Hopkins.

Surveys have shown that the two greatest fears in life are death and public speaking. I remember in school the feeling of dread as I sat in my seat, waiting to present my oral book report: my stomach churning, my mouth dry, my palms clammy.

What if I forgot what I was supposed to say? What if I mis-pronounced a word? What if I was horrible? All I wanted to do was melt into my chair and disappear.

I was too sad, too angry, and too tired to have these fears affect me now. The way I looked at it, I could share my inner-most thoughts with three hundred strangers, or I could get hit by a Mack truck—either way I would feel nothing. I knew I had to relive Josie's death for these strangers because the thought of her story never reaching beyond Hopkins was worse.

> "I am not looking for sympathy," I told the audience as I gripped the podium. "I just want you to fix this broken system, the system that let Josie and ninety-eight thousand other people down this year. You are the ones who can make these changes."

I squinted through the glaring lights to look into the eyes of three hundred brilliant doctors, nurses, and administra-tors from all over the country and tried, unsuccessfully, to hold the tears back.

Standing on the stage that day felt like a good grief-therapy session. I talked and they listened. Not only did they listen, but they showed me they cared. They stood up and applauded. As I walked off the stage, people shook my hand and said thank you. They hugged me as they whispered their own stories of medical errors in my ear: the loved ones they, too, had lost, and the mistakes they had witnessed at patients' bedsides. I did not cry alone that day.

I realized as I flew home that Josie's story had struck a chord with the very people who could fix the problem.

I could not stop thinking about their reaction, how they listened to me, how they cried and confided in me. They seemed hungry for something, though I wasn't sure what. Maybe it was the fact that I was coming at patient safety from a different angle. I wasn't talking about the data and statistics. I didn't have a lengthy PowerPoint presentation. I wasn't one of them: I was an outsider with a real story.

I was happy to be back home with the children and Tony. With four-year-old Eva on my lap I flicked on the computer and watched in disbelief as the e-mails poured in from doctors, nurses, and administrators who had been in the audience. They wanted copies of my speech to take to their hospitals and share with their fellow doctors and nurses.

A cancer doctor who was a leader of a patient safety non-profit organization had been in the audience and happened to have a video camera that day and had filmed my speech. His name was Dr. Charles Denham but people called him Chuck. A few days after the conference he sent me a box. I opened it and there they were: twenty DVDs of my speech, titled *Josie's Story* and with Josie's picture on each one. He told me to give them to any hospital that asked for one and in return I should suggest that they make a donation to the Josie King Foundation.

"What should I ask for, fifteen dollars, twenty dollars?"

"The health care industry is used to paying good money for educational videos," he told me. "Ask for $250. They will be happy to support the Josie King Foundation."

With each e-mail and DVD request came a story, usually from a nurse. They told me a little bit about themselves:

where they were from and at which hospital they worked. Some were mothers and some were new to nursing, but most had seen medical errors at the bedside. All of them thanked me for sharing Josie's story and told me that it had changed the way they cared for their patients. They wanted to use the film to inspire their fellow doctors and nurses.

A week later, I went to the post office with the twenty DVDs and shipped them to various hospitals around the country. Chuck sent me a box of forty more. Within days they, too, had been sent off. Slowly but surely, Josie's story was creeping beyond the walls of Hopkins and I was building personal relationships with doctors and nurses around the country.

13

As word spread through the health care industry about my speech in Boston, other speaking requests started coming in—from the National Patient Safety Foundation (NPSF), the Agency for Healthcare Research and Quality (AHRQ), and the Joint Commission. I had no idea who these groups were or what they did. I wasn't sure who to go to for advice, so I again called my onetime adversary Rick Kidwell.

He answered my questions and gave me a rundown on the players in the patient safety world, which, I was beginning to realize, was an industry unto itself.

He told me that if I could stand the mental anguish then I should talk to these organizations. "This whole concept of patient safety is complicated," he said. "It's a process of changing the culture and that is an extremely difficult thing to do because you have to change the way people have been trained to think and behave. Doctors and nurses get fed so much information on patient safety that they sometimes just glaze over it all."

He told me that they didn't want to hear it from him or from their peers. "Josie's story and the way you tell it is powerful. It inspires people to think about patient safety. They'll listen to you."

It was hard leaving the children and Tony. And I hated flying. I often wished Tony would tell me not to do it but, like Rick, he was always there to give me a gentle push. He told me this was what we needed to do for Josie. And when I looked to Gloria, she, too, nudged me out the door. "Get on out there girl," she told me.

I began realizing that the children actually liked it when I left. Tony took them to Miss Shirley's Café on the way to school, where they ordered strawberry pancakes with whipped cream. Gloria let them watch cartoons and eat ice cream when they came home from school. They did all the things that I never let them do during the week.

Like Rick, Dr. Pronovost was proving to be a valuable ally. He was an amazing public speaker, humble and charismatic. A few weeks after my speech in Boston, he and I spoke before the NPSF, the National Patient Safety Foundation, in Washington, DC. We talked about the need for a culture of safety in the health care industry. I spoke from a patient's perspective, Peter from an institutional perspective. We were a good team.

Soon after, I received a phone call from a producer who worked for the *Good Morning America* show. He wanted the two of us to appear on the show. Peter loved the idea, but Hopkins was hesitant. They had accepted the fact that I was talking about the hospital's mistakes to the health care industry, but they were not ready to share our intertwined story on national television.

"They won't let me," Peter said. "They're thinking that if I don't do it, you won't do it."

I called the Hopkins public relations officer, who proceeded to explain to me that, within the hospital, there was some reluctance for Peter to appear on the show because they did not think it was in the best interest of Hopkins' reputation.

I told her it wasn't about what was in the best interest for Hopkins. It was about preventing medical errors. "If Peter and I are on national television, maybe some doctors and nurses and families might be listening. Maybe they'll get the message that ninety-eight thousand people are dying every year and that someone better do something about it. We gave you money and now you're not helping me do what's right! Shame on you and shame on Hopkins," I said angrily. "I'll be sitting with Charlie Gibson next week and I would think Hopkins would look a heck of a lot better if someone from there was sitting next to me."

A week later, Peter, Tony, and I took a train to New York City. We were accompanied by a representative from the Hopkins public relations office, who treated us all to dinner the night before. She followed me closely, keeping a watchful eye and looking for signs of me as the loose cannon about to go off.

The next morning we arrived at the *Good Morning America* set. The lights were bright and the cameras pointed straight at us. I saw a photo of Josie flash above me on a screen. It was one of her wearing a dark blue shirt, smiling her one-toothed smile. Millions of people were seeing her face and about to hear our story.

It was a short interview, just a few minutes, and much of it was Peter telling Charlie Gibson what Hopkins was doing to prevent medical errors.

In the end, it was a nice publicity piece for Hopkins. They were pleased with themselves and although it made me cringe to see Hopkins enjoy the positive spin on the story, I knew that they had made a promise to become safer on national television, in front of millions of viewers.

After the show, Tony dashed off to work in his New York City office. I sat next to Peter on the train back to Baltimore. He worked on his laptop as I looked out the window, wishing that Josie was waiting for me at home with Jack, Relly, and Eva. I felt myself slipping. Peter must have sensed it because he closed his laptop and asked me when my birthday was.

"September fourth," I said, keeping my gaze toward the window, not wanting him to see my welling eyes. "When's yours?"

He told me his birthday was February 22.

Sometimes in life there are little coincidences, and sometimes those coincidences are signs, guideposts that say, *stop and pay attention, this means something.*

"That's the day Josie died," I said.

Peter and I both agreed that this was more than a mere coincidence. It had to be a sign, a sign that we were on the right track.

The more I worked with Peter, the more it became apparent to me that his CUSP program was a really good thing. His whole philosophy was to create change from the bottom up, empowering nurses and frontline staff to identify the problems and fix them themselves rather than being directed by upper management. One of the nice things about Peter's approach is that it creates ownership of the problem and gets everyone involved. Peter used to tell me that when it comes to patient safety there must be an equal-level playing field. There can be no hierarchy.

With all of the ideas that were being generated, projects that were being formed, and the lessons that were being learned I began thinking that perhaps CUSP should be made electronic so that other hospitals could benefit and share their stories—their lessons learned—with one another. I knew I didn't have the brains to put it together, and I knew it would cost thousands of dollars to get someone else to. My brother-in-law Jay was an educational software expert who had just sold his software company and was looking for a new project. I sent him everything I was learning about patient safety: books, articles, Web sites. I sent him the report *To Err Is Human.* I needed to convince Jay that this should be his next project. I needed to introduce him to Peter Pronovost.

A few months later, Peter and I were in Boston giving another IHI presentation. I invited Jay, who lived nearby, to check out the IHI scene and, more importantly, to join Peter and me for a drink in the hotel bar. I sat and watched while Peter and Jay connected. Peter's enthusiasm was contagious. Jay took it all in, listening while Peter talked at length about CUSP.

A week later, Jay flew down to Baltimore and the two of us spent the morning in Peter's office. There were folders with slips of paper, word documents, e-mails, and spread sheets. Information was scattered everywhere but Peter explained how it all worked and we were all in agreement: CUSP was great, but it was too cumbersome and took too much man-power. It needed to be electronic. Jay got to work and a year later, in collaboration with the Johns Hopkins Center for Innovation in Quality Patient Care, we formed the Patient Safety Group.

The Patient Safety Group would offer a Web-based project management tool that supported Peter's CUSP program, called eCUSP. No longer would patient-safety issues remain in a manila folder on someone's desk waiting to be read. And with the networking power of the Internet, hospitals now had a mechanism for sharing their efforts with others.

It was great to have Jay on board. He was smart, always had good advice, and, most of all, he was fun to work with. He was like an older brother to me and, like me, he quickly got immersed in the health care industry and realized the magnitude of our project.

He created the first JosieKing.org Web site, which incredibly simplified my life. Now hospitals, instead of calling me, could simply go to the Web site, download the transcript of my speech, or request a DVD. There was information about the Josie King Pediatric Patient Safety Programs at Hopkins and about the Patient Safety Group. People could also learn about the Josie King Foundation and read about patient safety. We were slowly making headway.

Before long the Patient Safety Group was up and running in hospitals throughout the country. The Josie King Foundation continued to receive donations from all over the world thanks to our DVD, which had now been translated into Hebrew and Spanish. The two Josie King Pediatric Patient Safety Programs that we had started at Hopkins were also doing well. We had had a sixth-month meeting at the hospital and it was nice to see firsthand that changes had been made and that things were progressing.

Dr. George Dover came to me with an idea. "What would you think if the Children's Center hired a person totally dedicated to patient safety? Their sole purpose would be to make sure people listen, communicate, and report patient-safety concerns."

I loved the idea. I knew it would make Hopkins safer, and I knew that if I could collaborate with this patient-safety person, Tony and I would feel even more comfortable that our donation was being used the right way.

Dr. Marlene Miller was a young pediatrician who had been working for AHRQ, doing research on patient safety and quality. I liked her from the start. She was a pediatrician and the mother of two young children. I also liked that she was married to Peter Pronovost. I imagined that their dinner conversations might revolve around patient safety and Hopkins. I knew that the two of them could make good things happen.

The Josie King Foundation gave Hopkins the money to hire Dr. Miller and she would report directly to Dr. Dover. It was clear to me that whatever safety concerns she or Peter had would be taken seriously at Hopkins.

14

My weekly grief sessions with Sandra Fink were going well. I was sticking with her recommendation to try new things and I was getting better at the guitar and had practically mastered "Edelweiss." I was learning how to live with my sadness. I could stand in front of a person, have a conversation, and appear to be somewhat normal. Trying new things forced me to get out of my grief a little bit and made the time go by. The painting, the sanding, the writing, they all forced me to concentrate on something other than my sadness.

We would sit down in her office and she would begin the session by asking me to tell her about Josie's burial. I knew this exercise by now. If you talk about something over and over again it helps you process it. So I talked, telling her every miserable detail. She asked if there were any pictures of Josie around the house. I told her there were not.

"I think you need to put some up," she said. "I think the children need to see that Josie is still a part of their lives."

Sometimes I looked at Sandra and hated her for telling me what to do when she had no idea what it felt like, the searing pain of seeing Josie's face, her smile, her snaggletooth, her cowlick—she had never lost a child. What was the purpose of having pictures of Josie around the house? Why make the pain worse? I decided I didn't want to talk about the burial and Josie's pictures anymore.

"What about having a baby?" I asked.

She looked at me, surprised, and gave me the lecture that she had given me so many times before when I had talked about finding a new home, a new husband, a new life. "Most therapists would agree that after a traumatic event like this, it's best to wait a full year before any major changes are made."

I had read the grief books and she was right. The books advise that after the loss of a child it is best not to make any life changes until after the first year. Don't move to a different house thinking that its new rooms will keep away the sad memories—the pain and sadness will follow you there. Don't move to another city thinking a fresh start will help—the pain and sadness will follow you there, too. And the thing the books stressed the most was don't have a baby right away thinking he or she will make the pain go away. A new baby cannot replace the child who has died. The pain and sadness will follow you wherever you go and whatever you do. Wait a year. You will think more clearly then.

Tony and I had all of those thoughts. We wanted to run away from it all but the reality had sunk in and we knew that no matter where we were or what we did Josie's loss would be felt forever.

"Well," I said, "I'm six months pregnant." I could tell she was surprised and didn't quite know what to say. After a few seconds she got up, came over, and hugged me.

Tony and I had never really talked about having another baby. We both knew that we could never replace Josie, but there was something we wanted. We wanted hope. We wanted a new beginning. Just like drinking water and eating food, I had to be pregnant in order to survive.

This pregnancy was nothing like the others. I didn't jump for joy when I missed my period and I didn't burst with happiness when the blue line appeared on the pregnancy test. I also didn't look forward to the monthly doctor appointments. In fact, I dreaded them. I hated sitting in the waiting room looking at all the other young mothers to be. I was different from them. We had nothing in common. I sat in the corner and hid behind *Time* magazine, staring at the words, trying to hold back the tears. I felt as if I were betraying Josie. Smelling the antiseptic and seeing the white coats, the metal trays, and the instruments sent my mind whirling back to the Hopkins PICU.

I was scared to death and, waiting for the doctor to come in, I would sit on the cold table in my paper gown and cry. I cried at every appointment. My doctor knew what to expect whenever she entered the room.

I took my vitamins and ate healthy food but, besides that, I blocked out the pregnancy completely. Tony and I hardly ever spoke about it. We both knew that until this baby came we had to continue to go through our work of grieving.

In the sixth month Tony's large T-shirts and sweaters could no longer hide my bulging belly. We had to tell people. One crisp sunny day, I cut through the neighbor's yard to go for a walk in the woods. She was working in her garden and said hello. She had a sad look on her face whenever she saw me and now she had tears in her eyes. We hadn't told anyone about my being pregnant, not even the children, but for some reason I felt like telling her. She threw her gloves in the air and hugged me. Just like that, she looked at me happily again, and as the weeks and months of pregnancy progressed, and as we began to tell our news to friends and family, all of the reactions were exactly the same.

I had gotten into the routine of walking in the woods once or twice a week with my friend Laura, who had bought her fiddle with me and who understood what it was like to lose a child. Misery loves company and I enjoyed hers and looked forward to our walks. She had asked me many times before about a baby shower, and each time I told her that I really and truly did not want one. I had never been much of a baby shower person, and certainly wasn't one now.

"I think I need to tell you something," she said one November morning as we walked along the trail. "When we get back to your house, there's going to be a little surprise baby shower for you. I don't want you to be too caught off guard, so that's why I'm telling you now, so you can try to act surprised."

And so I acted surprised when my friends and Gloria popped out from behind the sofa. They had brought Starbucks coffee, bagels, and fresh fruit. We sat there in the sunny kitchen, all of my friends who, for months, had struggled with me through my grief, and for a short while that day nothing felt awkward. We thought only about the future and this baby who would soon be arriving. They sat around me and handed me gift after gift. The last gift was from my friend Mary Ellen—not a gift for the new baby, actually, but gifts for Jack, Relly, and Eva: three little bears. Her note read:

When the Lord closes a door, somewhere he opens a window.
　—from *The Sound of Music*

I felt lucky to have friends who wanted to make me happy, if just for a moment. When they left, Gloria and I looked at the piles of gifts. She gathered them up, making various comments: "Won't this be nice if it's a boy," "We'll put this in the bassinet," and "I'll get one of the workmen to help me hang the mobile." I realized as I watched her in her excitement that this baby was coming very soon, and that maybe it was all right to start feeling happy about it. Maybe I could do both: I could grieve for Josie when it was time to grieve, and be happy for this new baby when it was time to be happy. Just like Mary Ellen's note said, a door had closed, but maybe it was time to crack open a window.

I was pretty good at childbirth. I had been through four and, with the exception of them all being a little early, nothing had ever gone wrong. So I was not prepared to be lying on a stretcher with doctors and nurses rushing me into the operating room because the baby was in distress. Tony held my hand and told me everything was going to be all right. He was as white as a sheet. As they put the gas mask on my face, I prayed to God that if this baby died, to please let me never wake up. I wasn't afraid to die as I lay there staring into the white light above me, smelling the fumes from the gas. The anesthesiologist held my head between his hands and wiped the tears from my face as the doctor sliced my insides apart to retrieve the baby whose heart rate was rapidly plummeting.

Samuel Mackall King was born on November 20, 2001, a perfectly healthy little boy who weighed seven pounds, eight ounces. When I held him in my arms for the first time my heart filled up like a balloon. Jack had always wanted a little brother and he showed up at the hospital with football cards in hand. Sam was born on Relly's sixth birthday, the best birthday present ever. She wanted to take him to school for show-and-tell. Four-year-old Eva just wanted to be the big girl and hold him in her arms like a baby doll. That day, as all six of us sat in my hospital room, this little boy made our heavy hearts light again.

When Sam was a baby I did not travel. While Jack, Relly, and Eva were at school I would set his bassinet next to my computer and research the world of medical errors as he slept. I kept a watchful eye on him, making sure he was breathing. I breast-fed him for eight months, making sure I gave him everything he needed to have a strong immune system.

As he grew into a toddler, he and I went to a "Mommy and Me" music class. I made sure that I washed his hands after each class so that he would not catch a cold that would turn into pneumonia, which would send us to the hospital, where he could develop a horrible infection and die. When we went to see the pediatrician for his one-year checkup, I held my breath, dreading a diagnosis.

That year, we faced our first Thanksgiving and Christmas without Josie. Although we had Sam to distract and amuse us, the pain of missing Josie was ever-present. When I looked into Sam's blue eyes, I marveled at how wonderful it was that he was completely clueless: he had no idea that he was coming into a broken family. I tried my best to talk more about Josie with the children. Sometimes I even put a picture of her on the table, as Sandra had suggested, but eventually the sight of her smiling face became too unbearable and I would put it away.

The children never said anything about the picture of Josie that would come and go from the family room table. I believe that their hearts, like mine, had filled with love for Sam, but that the sadness of missing Josie was still there.

Having Sam did not lessen my grief for Josie; it did not make the pain go away. I still wrote in my journal and sometimes I wrote to her, telling her how much Jack, Relly, and Eva missed her. I told her about Sam and how I wished they could have known each other. I told her how sorry I was that I had let this happen. But when Sam cried or woke up from a nap, I snapped into the present, putting my pencil down to wipe the tears away. He was the timer on my grief clock.

February 22, the second anniversary of Josie's death, loomed, and I dreaded it. In some respects the second year had been harder than the first. The shock had worn off and other people had moved on. We suffered alone. Tony and I decided that we needed to get away. We needed distraction, a diversion, so we rented a house in Deep Creek, a tiny ski resort in western Maryland. Knowing that this would be a hard weekend for us, my parents and my sister Margaret and her family joined us.

The morning of February 22, I sat alone in my room, looking out at the frozen lake as Sam slept in his crib. I listened to the children and their cousins downstairs in the kitchen, clattering about as Tom, Margaret's husband, and Tony made pancakes. I did not want to light a candle and I did not want to let a bouquet of helium balloons fly up to heaven.

I did not want to talk about her or look at her picture. All I wanted was for this horrible day to be over.

I turned on the television looking for something to keep me in the here and now, something to bring me back from reliving that day when I had sat and held Josie for the last time. Katie Couric would do. I listened to her deliver the news and one story catapulted me away from feeling sorry for myself.

". . . a young girl died from medical errors at prestigious Duke University Medical Center . . ."

I listened to Jesica Santillan's story unfold on national television. Jesica, a seventeen-year-old girl from Mexico with an enlarged and weakened heart and lungs that were not functioning properly, had come to the United States to receive treatment at Duke University Medical Center in Durham, North Carolina. She underwent a heart-lung transplant. Only toward the end of the surgery did the lead surgeon realize there had been a terrible mistake. Jesica's blood type was O, but the heart and lungs she had received were type A. Her body began rejecting the healthy organs soon after she received them and her health quickly deteriorated as Duke scrambled to find another set of organs. On February 20, she underwent a second transplant but complications quickly set in and she was too weak to recover. She died on February 22.

The news of the horrific medical mistake was on every major network. As I watched the footage of Jesica's mother, I wanted to reach out to her. There was no one else who could understand what she was going through. I wanted to help her.

I picked up the phone and dialed 411. I got through to Duke and after being transferred all over the hospital, I finally

ended up speaking with Dr. Karen Frush, the hospital's patient safety officer. She had heard of me and knew Josie's
story. I asked her if there was some way I could help Mrs.
Santillan. She told me it was too late. Mrs. Santillan had been
advised not to talk to anyone from the hospital, so there was
no way she could put me in touch with her. She told me that
the doctors and nurses who had taken care of Jesica wanted
desperately to reach out to Mrs. Santillan. I could hear the
sadness and resignation in her voice but the legal system had
taken over and Duke was bracing itself for a massive media
and legal onslaught.

If I couldn't help Jesica's mother, perhaps I could help
Duke. My mother once told me that when you're feeling sorry
for yourself the way to feel better is to help someone in need.
I told Dr. Frush about the changes that Hopkins had made
since Josie's death and I suggested that she talk to some of
the people from Hopkins.

That morning in Deep Creek, as I listened to the news of
Jesica's death and talked to Dr. Frush, I felt my misery subside. There was someone who needed me, something I had
to do. I began thinking how strange it was that Jesica died
of medical errors on the exact date that Josie had died. To
me this was more than a mere coincidence. It was a sign. I
had to pull myself together.

Sam woke up from his nap and I scooped him up as he
arched his back, stretching his arms and legs. I held his warm
little body against my chest, put on my slippers, and joined
the others for breakfast.

We got through the day by being together and staying
busy. My father lit a fire and we played games and read
books. Jack and his cousin Benjamin built a card house. Relly

and Eva and their cousins Sheila and Marlee soaked in the hot tub with my mother. Margaret and I took a long walk around the lake.

My mother had insisted on bringing venison up from Virginia to serve for dinner. All day Margaret and I eyed the frozen slabs of meat sitting on the counter. We had eaten our fair share of Big-Rel-needing-to-clean-out-the-freezer meals.

"What year do you think it's from?" I asked Margaret as she unwrapped a slab.

"I don't know, but I don't think it's from this year," she said, pointing to the freezer burn.

Tony and Tom had been in the family long enough to know the routine in Big Rel's kitchen. First of all, you always checked the date on the milk and yogurt. When it came to meat, especially game, someone other than Big Rel needed to take a look and it couldn't be Pop. He loved anything that he shot no matter how long it had been frozen—no matter how many times a storm had knocked out the electricity causing the meat to thaw and refreeze. He would fry it up in a stick of butter, pour some salt and breadcrumbs on it, add a little more salt, and then take a bite.

"Mmm mmm, this'll make your eyes pop out and your stomach say howdy," he'd say as we all watched. He'd take a swig of red wine and then go in for more.

Tony and Tom inspected the meat.

"We need to supplement," Tony said, as he began looking through the cabinets. He took out a bag of sun-dried tomatoes, a box of risotto, and a head of garlic and started to cook, while Tom opened a bottle of red wine and poured them each a glass.

As the hours ticked by, I kept slipping into the past—remembering to the minute exactly what happened on that February twenty-second—*The children were saying good-bye. Amal was listening to her heart. Tony and I were holding her*—and as the afternoon wore on I started slipping back into grief. I went up to my room and looked out the window. Margaret came in and stood next to me as we watched Big Rel and the children sledding.

"I wish Josie could be out there with them," I said.

She put her arm around my shoulder. "We just need to get through today," she said. "Tomorrow will be better." She walked over to the full-length mirror. "Come here. I want to show you something."

At five foot six, Margaret was the perfect height, not too tall, not too short. She had dark olive skin and eyes the color of brown sugar, but her greatest asset was her long, thick hair. It flowed straight down her back. My mother said it was the color of blackstrap molasses.

We were as close as two sisters could be and sometimes we even had the same dreams, the same thoughts. Unbeknownst to our husbands, we had planned our pregnancies together. We were more than sisters, we were best friends, and when Josie had been at the hospital Margaret stood by her side with me, giving me encouragement. And like only a sister could do, she made me laugh when I wanted to cry.

When Josie died Margaret stayed in Baltimore with me for days. After she had gone back home to DC, she called every few hours to check in on me. Each time she called I told her I was fine, not to worry, but she didn't believe me. She would drive up from Washington and as I sat alone in Josie's room she would pop her head in and say "Let's go for a walk in the woods." Sometimes I was just too sad to do anything with her, though, and I was no longer the sister she had once known. Our days of laughter together seemed gone forever. As hard as she tried to walk with me into the darkness of my grief we both realized that I had to do it alone. And so she sat with me for days, watching and waiting for time to take its course.

"You're gonna love this," she said, pointing to her chin as she leaned in toward the mirror.

I looked closely and there it was, a little black whisker half an inch long.

We erupted into laughter. She told me she had found it a week ago and had been going to pluck it, but left it because she knew it would make me laugh.

We laughed so hard we cried.

"Okay, I did my job. Now this sucker is outta here," she said, reaching for the tweezers.

I told her she had to leave it just a little longer. She had to show everyone downstairs.

"I walked through the streets of Georgetown with this just for you. I guess I can leave it one more day if it makes you laugh more."

We wiped our tears away and went downstairs.

We fed the children hamburgers and hot dogs and Margaret sat at the end of the table as they each examined her whisker. After they ate, we set them up with a movie in the living room and sat down to grown-up dinner. We all held hands like we always did and Pop said grace. He said a little prayer for Josie, and Tony gave my hand an it's-all-right-don't-cry squeeze. My mother served the venison and we all chewed and chewed and loaded our plates up with Tony's risotto.

The next morning the ground was covered with a sheet of ice and my parents decided to get an early start before the roads got worse. The rest of us decided to caravan and meet for lunch. Tony put the Suburban in four-wheel drive, giving it just enough gas to creep up the steep icy driveway. We waited and watched from above as the minivan tried to make it but it just spun its tires. We got out of the car and went down to help. We had no salt or sand, and it was too steep and slippery to push from behind.

The children stood on the side of the driveway, delighted that they could spend more time with their cousins, and watched as the grown-ups tried padding the wheels with newspaper, bits of wood, and gravel, anything to give the minivan some traction. Nothing worked. Tom and Tony went back into the house to look for something else to put under the wheels.

"What *is* that?" Margaret asked as we watched them emerge from the house carrying something red and brown lying on newspaper.

"I think it's the venison," I said.

We watched them lay the leftover, leathery slabs of meat under each wheel. Margaret got in the driver's seat as Tony, Tom, and I pushed from the sides. The wheels gripped the meat, crept over the ice, and up the hill as the children cheered. We piled into the cars and headed to our lunch destination, leaving the venison for a hungry fox.

We had made it through the weekend. We had made it through another year without Josie.

One of the ladies from the church group that I had briefly attended once told me that God was helping me.

"I don't feel God helping me," I responded.

She cupped her hands together as if she were holding a ball and said, "All of your friends, your family, people you don't even know are holding you up. They are helping you get through this. That is God."

That day as we drove home from Deep Creek I could feel my family holding me, my sister with her whisker, my mother with her home cooking, my father keeping the hearth warm. They were there that weekend to support us, to keep us from falling.

I called Marlene Miller first thing Monday morning and told her about my conversation with Dr. Frush. The two of them talked and soon thereafter Marlene flew to Durham to meet Dr. Frush and the medical staff at Duke. Hopkins was helping Duke through this difficult time and the two doctors would ultimately become friends. They would work together to achieve the same goal of improving patient safety. They would spread their work to other hospitals, sharing what they had learned at their own institutions.

Dr. Frush and I talked often during the weeks following Jesica Santillan's death. She told me that many of the doctors and nurses who had cared for Jesica were seeking counseling and participating in grief therapy sessions. Dr. Frush was very concerned that some of the best doctors and nurses would not continue to work because of the grief and pain they were feeling. They all wanted desperately to reach out to Mrs. Santillan. They wanted to tell her how sorry they were, but all communication had been shut down.

I had never thought much about the suffering of health care providers when a medical error occurs. I had been too consumed by my own misery to put myself in their shoes. But through Dr. Frush's eyes I began to understand and I felt sorry for them. They had spent their careers trying to help people and nobody had meant for Jesica to die. Nobody had meant for Josie to die either.

15

I received a call from Peter Pronovost. He asked if I would talk to a group of second-year medical students at Hopkins. I had never spoken to medical students and the thought of influencing their young minds seemed somewhat intriguing. It was a quick car ride and I would only be gone for two hours. I told Peter I would do it. He said that a reporter for the *Baltimore Sun* wanted to cover the lecture and he asked if I would mind her being there.

Peter didn't know that in my anger and grief during those months after Josie died, I had been fantasizing about destroying Hopkins through the media. I had gone so far as to call the *Baltimore Sun* and ask for the person who covered health care issues, but Paul Bekman's repeated advice kept coming back to me—"If we go to the media now, it will just be a sad story, and then it will be old news." I would hang up before I spoke to anyone.

The settlement had been signed, the case had been closed, and I had stayed away from the media. And now Peter was unknowingly handing me what I had been wanting for so long: a reporter who was ready to write.

But I no longer cared. A part of me had moved on. I was busy working with Hopkins and other hospitals. I was sharing Josie's story and I was seeing the effect it was having on people. Something had changed in me. My obsession with the destruction of Hopkins had transformed into an obsession with the construction of a safer Hopkins, a safer health care industry. I no longer wanted to fight.

I thought about what Paul Bekman had said and I wondered if perhaps this reporter could help me reach my new goal: raising awareness and fixing the problem.

I arrived at the lobby of the building where I would be giving the lecture and saw Peter chatting with the reporter, Erika Niedowski. She looked exactly how I had imagined a newspaper reporter. She was in her mid-twenties, carried a black messenger bag slung across her back, and held a small notebook in her hands. She was pretty in a natural sort of way. I imagined her spending many late nights at the paper, writing and surviving on coffee.

As we took the elevator up she and Peter laughed and chatted as if they were old friends, he telling her about the amazing things that were going on at Hopkins. I stood there trying to act impressed and quickly became annoyed with myself for agreeing to meet with this reporter who seemed already to be on Hopkins' side. I wondered if she had any clue as to what Peter's almighty institution had done to my daughter.

I wanted to get out of the dingy gray elevator, away from Peter and Erika and their small talk. When the doors opened, I quickly walked to the bathroom, trying to hide my tears. I splashed water on my face and looked in the mirror. How could I have been so stupid? I reached under my brown sweater and pulled out the little gold locket that my father had given me a few weeks earlier. It was warm from my skin.

"You don't see lockets anymore," he had said as he handed it to me. He told me my great-grandmother had worn one after her son Jack died. "She said it kept him near to her heart." Jack had died in 1918, when the Spanish influenza was wiping out small towns across the country. Most streets in the city of Richmond had been quiet as parents kept their children inside, away from the deadly germs; public pools shut down and movie theaters closed. But unbeknownst to his parents, sixteen-year-old Jack, a Boy Scout, had been sneaking out at night to help transport the very sick to and from the hospital. His parents never fully recovered from his death.

As a young girl sitting in church, wedged between my mother and grandmother, I often looked up to the row of stained glass windows. There was one of my great-uncle Jack, kneeling, looking up at a bright light.

I daydreamed about this boy, Jack, wondering what he had been like. Had he had a girlfriend? What sports did he like to play? Was he funny like his sister, my grandmother? And the thing I wondered most: would I have risked my life for others the way he had?

I liked the round disk of locket that felt silky smooth in my hand. I imagined the fingers of a grieving mother from many years ago, rubbing it over and over again.

I opened the locket and looked at the smiling picture of Josie on the beach. The jeweler had placed the lock of hair not on the other side of the locket as I had expected, but on top of her head. It looked awkward, as if she were wearing a hat. I snapped the locket shut and let it slip down under my sweater, now chilly against my skin.

I sat in the audience while Peter introduced me. Erika was in the back taking notes. I stood up, walked to the stage, and began telling Josie's story. I could see it happening. The students stopped fidgeting, they put their pens down, and they closed their books and stared at me wide-eyed as I continued to speak. Josie's story was reaching into their hearts. Before I stepped away from the podium I asked the audience if they had heard of the IOM report *To Err Is Human*.

I stood waiting. Not a single person raised their hand.

I explained to them what the Institute of Medicine report had concluded in 2000, that between forty-four thousand and ninety-eight thousand people die every year from medical errors. "So, it's not just about this one story. It's about thousands and thousands of people who die every year." I asked if they talked about medical errors in school. A student raised his hand and told me that no one had ever talked to them about medical errors. "There was a mention of it once in an ethics class, but that was about it."

I walked off the stage and sat next to Peter while the next speaker began his presentation. I was rattled by the fact that these future doctors were taught how to cure diseases and mend broken bones, but they knew practically nothing about the fourth leading cause of death. I leaned over to Peter and whispered in his ear, asking why this wasn't in the curriculum.

"I don't know, but it's true," he whispered back. "That's why we need to keep at this. It's good that they hear from us."

At the end of the session, a few students came up to thank me. They told me that Josie's story had been one of the most eye-opening hours of medical school. "I'll never forget Josie's story," one of them told me. "It'll be with me for the rest of my career."

I stepped out into the cool afternoon, glad to be out of the conference room and on my way home. I was frustrated that these students weren't being exposed to the topic of medical errors. It almost seemed as if it was being kept a secret. The problem of medical errors was even bigger than I had thought. It wasn't just lurking in the hospitals, it was germinating in the medical schools and in the nursing schools.

I was heading to the parking lot when I saw Erika running toward me, clutching her notebook. She told me she was sorry about Josie and asked if I would spend some time with her next week. "Maybe we could have lunch and talk for an hour or two," she suggested.

"What, to talk about this presentation? We can just do that over the phone," I said a bit sharply, still annoyed with her for being so wowed by Hopkins. She told me she wanted to write an in-depth article on medical errors centered around Josie and Hopkins and the partnership that had been formed between us.

I stood there that chilly afternoon and listened to her. My conversation with Paul Bekman flashed back to me. This would be more than a sad story.

Erika and I met the next week, and the week after that and the week after that, talking for hours and hours. She asked questions and I answered. She came to our house and met Tony and the children. She read my journal. She studied Josie's medical records and death certificate. She followed me to conferences and meetings. She was becoming a part of my world, always listening, always writing.

I liked Erika and I liked her company. We were becoming good friends and as I was learning the ins and outs of the health care industry, so was she. Every day we seemed to learn something new and every day we were further amazed by the magnitude of the problem. She was also spending time at Hopkins on her own and would sometimes call me, frustrated that a certain doctor or nurse who had cared for Josie had refused to talk to her. She was getting the story only from the public relations department and that was not enough.

I picked up the phone and called the PR office and urged them to encourage the doctors and nurses to cooperate with Erika. "You've got to trust me on this," I told them. "It's not going to be a slaughter piece. It will raise awareness. In the end, I promise, this article will be a good thing for Hopkins."

I realized that I was promising Hopkins something that I really had no control over. Even though I trusted Erika, I was not 100 percent sure that the article wouldn't blow up on us all, ruining the relationships and trust for which I had worked so hard.

I was concerned for Hopkins but also for my family. I knew all of the old wounds would be reopened. People would look at us again as they had for the weeks and months after Josie died, with sadness in their faces, saying, "Oh there's that poor family." However, the potential good far outweighed our desire to protect our privacy.

One by one, Erika got her interviews. With each she would give me updates, and with each update I was learning something new about the people who had contributed to Josie's death. I was seeing the other side of the story—how Hopkins had been affected by Josie's death.

She told me that her interview with Chuck Paidas had gone well and that he had been very emotional when he spoke of Josie. At the end of the interview Chuck had walked over to his bookshelf and handed Erika *Corelli's Mandolin,* the book that I had given him, and showed her the inscription.

Dr. McKee had moved to New Haven and was working at Yale. Erika told me that she had spoken of Josie's case in great detail, spending hours answering Erika's questions and at times also becoming emotional.

With some detective work Erika was able to find the traveling nurse who had given Josie the methadone. A man had answered the phone when Erika called and told her that Brenda did not want to talk about it.

I wondered what had happened to this nurse and I wanted to know her side of the story. I wanted to know why she had given Josie the methadone. Sometimes I thought about asking Erika for her address and considered driving by her house to catch a glimpse of her or talk to her, but I never did.

Erika tried again and again to arrange an interview with the pain management doctor but was unsuccessful each time. Eventually, she was able to conduct the interview, but it did not go well. The doctor clearly did not want to talk about Josie's case.

Not long after Josie had died, Amal Murarka and his family moved to Chapel Hill, North Carolina, where he started a new job at the UNC Health Care. I had recently called him to tell him about Erika's project. He told me he would talk to her and proceeded to tell me about a training session that he and the other new employees of UNC Health Care had been required to attend.

"I sat there in a huge auditorium with a hundred doctors and nurses," he told me. "As I watched the video I realized that the woman speaking on the screen was you. It was you telling Josie's story." He said, "It was as if I was in the hospital room with you again, reliving that horrible day."

Amal had been a part of Josie's healing and then her death. He had witnessed what I had and the bond I felt with him was like no other. I had wanted him to remain a part of my life or at least I wanted to know that he was out there. I was happy that he and I had reconnected. He told me that he wanted to help me bring my patient-safety message to other hospitals in the North Carolina region. I knew Erika's interview with him would be a good one.

Three weeks later, on a hot muggy August day, Tony, the kids, and I returned home from our summer vacation. Jack, Relly, and Eva ran into the air-conditioned house as Tony yelled for them to come back and get their bags. I took Sam out of his car seat, grabbing whatever McDonald's Happy Meal trash I could reach. I was anxious to call Erika to hear how her interview with Amal had gone but as I prepared to call her the phone rang. It was Peter Pronovost. I took the phone outside where it was quiet.

"I don't know how to tell you this," he said. "Amal died last week."

It was hot outside and my mouth was dry. I felt shaky and sick to my stomach. I sat down on the stone steps.

He told me it had been a car accident. A tire blew and he lost control. His wife was in the car behind him. "They said he died instantly."

I hung up the phone and put my hands against the cool damp stone. I wanted to lay my face on the coldness, close my eyes, and have this all go away. I could hear the slow pulsing buzz of the cicadas getting louder and louder. I thought about his wife and two young daughters. I thought about his mother and father. Just like that, this wonderful man, this wonderful doctor, was gone.

Erika would later tell me that she had spoken to Amal just a few days before he died. She told me that Josie had made an impact on his life and his medical career. I wished that I could have told him how much he meant to me.

After a year of reporting, the *Baltimore Sun* ran Erika's two-part series. She had done an excellent job and, just as I had promised, Hopkins came out looking good.

The day after the first article appeared, I opened the paper to see a huge photo of Josie, with letters to the editor below it. A woman who ran a day care center out of her house suggested that I be put in jail for child abuse. A part of me had known this was going to happen. I didn't care. My skin was now as thick as leather and nothing else could cause me pain.

As I had suspected, the article did open old wounds. The condolence letters and the flowers poured into the house again, except this time they were from complete strangers. The man at the coffee shop who made hot chocolate for the children and the dry cleaner where Tony dropped his shirts had had no idea that our family had suffered such a tragedy, and now they didn't know what to say. It was as if Josie had died all over again. Ultimately, though, the article had raised awareness about medical errors and tens of thousands of *Baltimore Sun* readers now knew about the Josie King Foundation. That was all I cared about.

16

A few weeks after the article ran in the *Sun,* I received a letter from the pain management doctor at Hopkins who had refused to talk to Erika.

Dear Sorrel,

I am the anesthesiologist and pain specialist who ordered the methadone before Josie's death. This is one of the hardest letters I have ever written, but you need to know more of the story.

Before I start, I have to let you know that I cannot begin to tell you how sorry I am. I think of Josie often, with tears in my eyes. I saw Josie on rounds at about 11:00 a.m. I was shocked at how sick she looked. I had seen her before in the ICU. Her eyes were sunken, she was lethargic. I noticed particularly that she had very deep and frequent respirations. You might or might not remember that I listened to her with my stethoscope to see whether she had signs of a respiratory infection. I knew she had been febrile. She was not congested and her chest was completely clear. Being an anesthesiologist, I am trained to look for these subtle signs and come up with a differential diagnosis. I thought that she possibly had a metabolic acidosis with a respiratory compensation. I discussed this with the surgical resident who had just come into the intermediate care unit and told him that sepsis and dehydration can cause this kind of picture. But he did not agree with me.

As I was still very concerned, I went to look for Dr. McKee. I explained to her what I had seen and inquired whether blood for electrolytes or a reinsertion of a central line should be considered. Dr. McKee was very worried about reinserting the central line because of positive blood cultures before. We also talked about the methadone. I was concerned that Josie would withdraw after having received opioids for so long. Symptoms of opioid withdrawal include low-grade fevers and diarrhea. Having had diarrhea in the days before, I did not think Josie could tolerate a worsening of these symptoms. I had to make a decision: cutting the dose in half appeared to be the safest option. It would prevent withdrawal and prevent sedation, which we did not want.

When Josie arrested I was stunned. I felt, and still feel, that I had failed her and you. It was not the methadone. I had reached the decision to write the order using the best of my knowledge and experience. I have taken care of children with pain for more than ten years. Believe me, I have searched the whole literature to see whether I was completely wrong in writing the order. Could she have even absorbed the drug before the arrest? I considered all possibilities. What has been on my conscience was the fact that I saw how sick she was. I considered all possible diagnoses but I could not persuade people to listen to me. What should I have done? Take her in my arms and rush her back up to the PICU? People at Hopkins assured me that I had done everything I could. It was not enough.

I read the story in the *Sun,* though it was very difficult to do. I could not sleep this weekend and my children asked me what was wrong.

I have been an advocate for children all my life. I love my job. I have seen tragedy, and sick children where I tried my best and still the outcome was bad. Josie was different. I will never forget her.

The Webster's dictionary defines the verb *to forgive* as "to give up resentment against or the desire to punish; pardon." I didn't understand this concept when the preacher first brought it up to me a month after Josie died.

In October of 2006, a man walked into an Amish schoolhouse in Nickel Mines, Pennsylvania. He tied up eleven young girls and shot them in the head, one by one. Five of the girls died and the others suffered severe wounds. Within a week the media were reporting that the Amish people had forgiven this man for killing their children. A grandfather of one of the murdered girls was reported to have said to his family, "we must not think evil of this man."

I tried hard to understand how the Amish could feel this way, but I couldn't. Had they found some source of enlightenment that was beyond anything I could ever possibly comprehend? Or were they simply better people than I?

That day, as I read the letter from the anesthesiologist, I was finally able to step out of my own sadness and into someone else's. I realized for the first time that it was not just me who had been affected by Josie's death. Every nurse and every doctor who had cared for Josie had been changed by the experience.

In most cases such as Josie's, medical errors are not the result of one misplaced decimal point, one nurse, or one doctor. Usually it is a breakdown in the system, a breakdown in communication. Health care professionals are terrified of system breakdowns. They are terrified that they might be the one at the end of the line who administers the drug with the wrong dosage or signs off on a treatment that is given to the wrong patient. For any one patient, the number of potential errors that can occur is tremendous. Sometimes these errors happen and don't cause harm. Other times, errors occur, one on top of the other, leading to serious harm or death.

Peter Pronovost used to explain it to me in a simple way. "We call it the Swiss cheese effect. There are many holes, potential places for errors to get through. When all the holes line up, the errors get through the system and the patient dies."

One day, as I was walking up from the woods past the neighbor's house, I heard the loud ringing of the fire alarm that the workmen had been testing. As I came to the top of the hill I saw Laurie, a Hopkins nurse who was house-sitting for the neighbor, carrying two huge buckets of water, sloshing them all over her legs as she ran toward our house. I took in the sight of her and imagined her single-handedly putting out the fire. I called out to her. She turned around, looked at me, and then at the house.

"They're working on the alarm," I yelled. She put the two heavy buckets of water down.

"Thank God," she said, catching her breath.

I reached her. "You were going to go into that house and put out the fire, weren't you?" We looked at each other and laughed.

I had met Laurie the summer before Josie died. The four children and I were swimming at the neighbor's pool where she was house-sitting. I sat with Josie on my lap as she threw a little plastic gray shark in the water for Jack, Relly, and Eva to dive for. Laurie told me she was getting her nursing degree from Hopkins and was considering pediatric oncology as her specialty.

Months later, the little girl she had met wearing a pink bathing suit with yellow flowers would die of medical errors at the very hospital that was training her. Our paths would not cross for some time. My life had changed dramatically, and I had forgotten about her, but Laurie had not forgotten about Josie and me. Every day she went to work she was reminded of us. People were walking down the halls of Hopkins talking about Josie King, the little girl who died from medical errors on the seventh floor, and the question that rang through everyone's head was *how*? How could this have happened at Johns Hopkins?

Laurie and I ran into each other a while after Josie died and struck up a friendship. As I was beginning to find my way into the health care industry and the world of patient safety, Laurie was diving deeply into the world of pediatric oncology. She was passionate about patient safety, too, and she shared with me how, as a teenager, she had read an article about medical errors. She was shocked to learn that the health care industry made mistakes, mistakes that sometimes killed people. "That article," she said, "opened my eyes and set the patient-safety framework in my head." But it was Josie's death that would transform her into the ever-vigilant patient-safety driven nurse she would become.

I was fascinated by her life as a pediatric oncology nurse. She shared with me the happy stories and the miracles of medicine, and the sad stories, of which there were many.

"Wouldn't working in a maternity ward be more uplifting?" I suggested.

She looked at me and paused. "But, there's laughter," she said. "We play and have fun." She told me the children were resilient and inspirational. "Every day they make me smile."

"But Laurie," I asked, "when they die? How can you stand it?"

"Because every day I have the opportunity to help make things a little less stressful, a little less painful for these children and their parents."

Laurie often told me of the potential errors that she sometimes saw, usually on paper: a wrong dosage, a misplaced decimal point. She believed full-heartedly in the importance of reporting them, because if errors are not reported they cannot be fixed, but the existing culture made it very hard to report these errors. "I know it's the right thing to do," she said, "but it's hard."

In 2003, a five-year-old girl named Brianna Cohen was being treated for a brain tumor at the Hopkins Children's Center. She had received a bone marrow transplant and had been discharged from the hospital to recover at home. Part of her home care involved receiving intravenous feedings under the supervision of Johns Hopkins home-care unit.

One day after Brianna was infused with a solution bag, she became unresponsive. Her parents rushed her to the closest hospital but it was too late. On December fourth, Brianna died. Hopkins took full responsibility for her death.

Tests showed that the solution she had received had levels of potassium five times higher than the prescribed dose, thus causing her heart to stop. Further investigations revealed that the solution bag had not been mixed properly. In addition, Hopkins acknowledged that poor communication between hospital staff and pharmacy staff contributed to her death. Once again, poor communication had played a part in a system failure that had resulted in the death of a child.

Laurie and I talked soon after the news had broken. She was deeply saddened by Brianna's death and was shaken by the fact that the system she worked in every day and trusted had broken. "The system is so complex, with so many parts, so many people. But we trust each other," she said. "We must rely on each other to be excellent." She was afraid, not so much of making a mistake that she could have avoided, but of being the one at the end of the line, where all of the errors align and death occurs. "The thought of becoming a caterer is very tantalizing," she told me. "It's okay if mistakes are made when you're a cook. No one gets hurt."

Although she considered it, Laurie would never give up taking care of her kids with cancer. "They are my life," she told me. But not a day goes by where she is not constantly checking, double checking, and triple checking for mistakes, and doing whatever she can to prevent the tiniest of incidents from becoming an error and causing harm.

I've met hundreds of nurses who, like Laurie, are passionate about patient safety. I've listened to them teach a room full of health care providers how to make their hospital safer; I've sat next to them at large patient-safety conferences and

I've watched them at work in hospitals all around the country. Sometimes I meet them for only a brief moment, in a conversation, an e-mail, or an embrace. But each nurse who has heard Josie's story and whose hand I have shaken I believe has let her into their heart. They tell me that every time a patient asks a question or a mother says "something isn't right," they remember Josie.

I have come to accept the fact that as long as humans are involved, the system can break and mistakes will happen; however I know that there are nurses out there, thousands of them, who will do whatever it takes to keep their patients safe so that they can say, "not on my watch."

The more I thought about the doctors and nurses at Duke, Hopkins, and around the country who had been affected by medical errors, the more curious I became. Where do they go? Who do they talk to? How do they cope?

I asked Rick Kidwell these questions one day as we waited for an elevator. He told me that when a doctor or nurse has been involved in a medical error they go to the risk manager, someone like him. "If I think they are going to do something crazy, like jump out a window, I'll send them to someone else."

I was fairly certain he did not have a counseling or psychology degree. I thought about the doctors and nurses at Duke. I thought about the pain management doctor and the pain and guilt she had been living with for so long. Shouldn't she, shouldn't *they,* have someplace to go for help and support, a place where they could talk to other doctors and nurses who had been through something similar, a place where trained professionals were on hand to help them deal with their emotions and get them back on track.

The Hopkins pain management doctor inspired me with the notion that the Josie King Foundation needed to do something to help health care providers cope when there has been an unexpected event. Too often, the nurses, doctors, and other health care providers involved in medical errors are treated almost as forgotten victims. They are expected to return to work, return to the same conditions. They are expected to do so without talking about what happened, or only with talking about it to the hospital's risk management or legal staff.

In time, we would create a program called Care for the Caregiver, in which the Josie King Foundation funded a research project to look for ways to help doctors and nurses who had been involved in a medical error cope. But when I first read the pain management doctor's letter, there was one thing I knew I could do.

I wrote back to her and asked that she move on with her life and let go of Josie. She should stop feeling sad and guilty. I never thought I could have said that to the people who took Josie from me, but somehow the words came out. Looking back I realize that finally, without searching, I had found what it meant to forgive. It just happened. It felt natural, and it made me feel better.

17

Although I desperately wanted to change the system, I was beginning to resent the hospital work I was doing. I was spending too many days packing my children's lunches, taking them to school, hightailing it to the airport to hop on a flight where I sat white knuckled and sweating until the plane landed safely, then speaking to an audience of strangers, reliving Josie's horrible death, and racing back home to kiss the children good night. No longer therapeautic and constructive, the work was becoming destructive, and the travel was taking its toll on me.

One late night I was wandering around the short-term parking lot at BWI airport in the freezing cold, clutching my cell phone, ready to call 911 if a murderer jumped out of the shadows. I finally found my car, got in, locked the doors, blasted the heater, and sped toward the exit sign. I turned the radio on for company and felt the heat warm my aching cold feet that had been stuffed into uncomfortable high heels all day. The car was exactly how I had left it: my coffee cup still had coffee in it from the morning, Sam's cheese nips were still scattered on the floor from the day before, and Eva's library book sat, once again, forgotten on the back seat.

As I merged onto I-95 I thought about the children and wondered how their day had gone. I let my mind drift back to where I had been that day and began piecing together the events that had taken place. I replayed conversations I had had with doctors and nurses, trying to process all that I had seen, all that I had learned. My body guided the big Suburban but my mind was miles away as I sped down the dark highway. I stopped at a red light, looked around, and realized I had absolutely no idea where I was. All I knew was that I was not in a very safe-looking neighborhood. I picked up my cell phone and called Tony.

"What do you mean, you're lost? You're on 295 aren't you?"

"I don't think so. The only sign I see is Kenilworth Avenue and I don't think it's the Kenilworth Mall in Baltimore."

"Kenilworth Avenue? My God, you're in Washington, DC," he said.

As he guided me home, I could hear the children in the background asking him, "Did Mom get lost again?"

"Yes, Mom got lost," he replied.

Mom is always getting lost, I thought as I sped north on the highway with tears streaming down my face, furious at myself for being so stupid. I told Tony between exhausted, delirious sobs that I hated it. I hated it all and I was going to quit.

That Christmas I got the best present from Tony and the children that I could ever ask for: a Garmin, the global positioning system navigational device.

"Dad says you'll never get lost again if you use this," Jack said, and the children crowded around me as I opened the little box.

Never get lost again, I thought, *what a wonderful gift. What a wonderful, genius, clever, little invention.*

"Wherever you are, all you have to do is push the HOME button," Tony said. "You'll always know where to go."

Tony knew that beyond my getting lost traveling from one destination to another, I often just felt lost in general, lost without Josie, lost as I tried to find my way around the health care industry. As I held the little device in my hand I realized that his gift was another way in which he was going to help me find my way.

Another time, I was in a plane high above Chicago, heading home after a long day at Ascension Health. I was thinking about Tony and the kids and was looking forward to getting home. Thirty minutes after takeoff the pilot came on the intercom and told us that they were having some mechanical difficulties. The takeoff flaps seemed to be stuck and it was not safe to continue on. "We'll be heading back to O'Hare. Please prepare yourself for what might be a rough landing, and please remain calm."

I looked around at the other passengers for signs that perhaps I had misinterpreted what the pilot had just said. People who moments before were reading their books, listening to their iPods, or chatting with their neighbors were now nervously looking out the windows or at each other. They were tightening their seat belts. I looked up and down the aisle for the stewardess. I wanted desperately to hear that glorious snap and fizz of Coke cans opening but the aisles were empty. No trolley cart. No stewardess. I began to panic. I needed someone to talk to. With eyes tearing up, I turned to the man next to me.

He was an older man in his sixties, wearing a dark gray suit, and he had a *Wall Street Journal* in his lap. He reassured me, explaining that things like this happen sometimes. "Don't worry," he told me. "These pilots are good. They can land these planes no matter what goes wrong."

I asked him if he would hold my hand and talk to me while the plane landed.

He opened his hand and we talked about where we were from and where we were going. If he remained calm, I thought, then everything would be okay. I locked my eyes onto his, looking for signs of panic.

"Flight crew, prepare for landing, and everyone, please brace yourselves," the pilot said.

I moved closer to my new friend and concentrated on his every word, our foreheads almost touching. When he lifted his window shade, we could see the lights of Chicago getting closer. He asked me how many children I had and how old they were. I tried to concentrate on giving him answers, but all I could think about was how I wished I had told them I loved them one more time before I left. We could see the fire trucks and ambulances poised along the runway, ready to rescue us from a fiery blaze.

"Dear God, please just let this plane land safely. Don't make my children suffer any more loss," I thought. I could hear a woman a few seats in front of me crying as the plane slowly descended. I squeezed my friend's hand as we looked out the window.

The plane touched down: it was a perfect landing. We all clapped and cheered for the pilots.

An hour later, we boarded another flight to Baltimore. I sat with my new friend. We ordered wine and ate our pretzels together, chatting and laughing as if we had known each other for years. I silently vowed to never leave the children again.

*   *   *

It was neither the first nor the last time that I swore to end my travels and stop speaking at hospitals around the country but, as always, I returned home to e-mails from the doctors and nurses who had been in the audience and had been moved by Josie's story. They told me they were inspired to listen better, to communicate better. I decided that I would not immediately quit entirely: I would simply fulfill the speaking engagements that I had already committed to, and then that would be it.

While I was at a patient-safety conference in Florida talking to a doctor, I told him that this would probably be my last trip. The travel was getting to be too much. He told me he had a game plan for me, some ideas that might make me reconsider.

"You need to be selective," he said. "Don't accept every single speaking request. If the audience is under 250 people, don't do it. If you can't get a direct flight and if you can't be in and out the same day, don't do it." He asked me what my honorarium was.

An honorarium? Feeling like an idiot I told him I didn't even know what an honorarium was.

"An honorarium is a speaker's fee," he explained. "Every speaker here is getting paid. Not only is this part of their job, but they're also receiving extra money for these speeches."

I told him that I didn't feel comfortable taking money. "I think it's just something I have to do."

"You don't have to take the money," he said. "They can send the honorarium to the Josie King Foundation. You tell any organization that wants you to speak that they need to make a donation. That way you are doing what you need to do *and* making money for your foundation."

He also told me that there was no reason I should be driving myself to and from the airport. "They will cover *all* of your expenses, including transportation to and from the airport. Hire yourself a driver," he told me.

My eyes lit up. I loved this idea. "But I still have to relive Josie's death over and over again, and I'm tired of doing that," I told him.

"People need to hear the story," he said, "but I also think they'd be interested in hearing about all the work you've been doing with the foundation. Why don't you start focusing the talks more on those accomplishments? Tell them all of the good that has come from Josie's death. Inspire them to do the same."

Throughout the rest of the day I thought about what he had said. Josie's story *was* becoming more than the story of a horrible tragedy. Her death had inspired change, real change. The foundation was growing and amazing things were happening. Yes, he was right. *That* was what I wanted to talk about.

I hired a friendly driver named Ron and after that there was a bit more pep in my step as I walked out my front door to get into his maroon sedan and be driven to the airport.

My message changed, also. I no longer focused solely on Josie's death. I talked about the foundation's projects and programs and, while I had the attention of change makers, I began spinning other topics into my speech, one of which was disclosure.

"It's not about the money," I told audiences. "It's about telling us the truth, apologizing and fixing the problem. There may well be a lawsuit. But by doing the right thing, families might give back to the hospital that harmed them, if it means no one else will be hurt." I said this over and over, in front of thousands of health care providers, hoping that maybe, just maybe, they would get the message and treat their patients and families the way Hopkins had treated us.

With my new strategy for managing my work and travel, Tony and I decided that I should continue talking to hospitals and industry leaders. I went to Chicago, New York, Boston, Washington, DC, Charlotte, Nashville, and London. Always in and out as quick as possible. The trips were thrilling and I was meeting fascinating people and seeing amazing hospitals. Sometimes, though not often, I was still left frustrated.

The Cleveland Clinic invited me to speak and it was an easy flight. They were making a donation, and they were one of the biggest and most renowned health care institutions in the world. There was one glitch—I'd be missing Jack's eleventh birthday. Tony, Jack, and I talked it over and decided that Jack could have two family celebrations: one on his real birthday, without me, and another the next night, with me.

It was early March and, when the plane landed in Cleveland, a snowstorm was just beginning to kick up. I was annoyed with myself for leaving Jack on his birthday and potentially getting snowed in, and also for not having enough sense to wear a warm coat. The only bright side was knowing that I would finally meet Dr. Karen Frush in person. Karen and I had spoken many times since that first phone call I had made to her after the death of Jesica Santillan, but we had never met in person. That evening she and I would present together.

The Cleveland Clinic has been ranked as one of the top four hospitals in the country by the *U.S. News and World Report*. It has made huge contributions to the world of medicine, including identifying carpal tunnel syndrome, developing the kidney dialysis machine, linking high blood pressure to heart disease, and greatly refining heart bypass surgery. But most impressive of all is the Cleveland Clinic's breakthrough work in the field of cardiology. Fourteen years in a row, it was rated as the best heart hospital in the country. Some say it is the best in the world. Kings from far-away countries, Arab sheikhs, world leaders, and movie stars all travel here to be treated by the fine doctors and nurses who make up the Cleveland Clinic.

As the driver made his way through the snowy streets of Cleveland, he told me that this hospital was so enormous that a hotel was connected to it. "An Arab sheikh who was here for treatment paid for his entire family to stay in the penthouse for months. The sheikh was so pleased with his treatment that he gave each doctor and nurse a Rolex watch. No doubt about it," he said proudly, "this place is the best."

I looked out the window at the enormous gray buildings, one after the other. "Forty buildings covering a hundred and forty acres," the driver told me. It seemed like a city in itself. He pointed to the hotel, "That's where you'll be meeting the others, Dr. King."

Dr. King, I liked the sound of that, but I told him I was not a doctor.

"What are you then?"

I paused. "I don't really know what I am. I guess I'm just a person who tries to inspire hospitals to be safer."

With marble floors, high ceilings, and fresh cut flowers, the Cleveland Clinic seemed the perfect place for an Arab sheikh to stay. I was greeted in the lobby by a friendly woman who informed me that I would be joining some executives for lunch and then would be given a tour of the hospital.

I followed her as she wove through the tables. The restaurant was darkly lit, with green leather chairs, white tablecloths, and baskets of bread on each table.

Karen Frush recognized me and waved. She walked around the table to greet me. She was a tall woman, and striking, her brown bangs and high cheekbones perfectly framing her warm, blue eyes. She didn't look like an ER doctor; I imagined her instead in a Chanel suit, running a fashion magazine in New York City.

We ordered our meals and I listened as Karen and the other doctors told me about their various patient-safety efforts.

Karen's viewpoint for patient safety was unique. She had been a nurse before going back to medical school to become an ER doctor, and she had a commanding presence at the table. Not only did she seem like the perfect person to be running patient-safety programs at Duke, she seemed like the perfect person to be traveling to other hospitals, spreading the word. Nurses as well as physicians would be drawn to her.

After lunch, Karen and I were given a tour of the hospital. I had been on quite a few hospital tours, but this massive complex was unlike anything I had ever seen. We traveled through the hospital on moving walkways that took us from one concourse to another. The long hallways had street names and posted at various points were maps with red arrows telling us exactly where we were.

As we moved through the hospital Karen and I chatted. She told me about the patient-safety work she was doing at Duke and at other hospitals around the country. Her greatest challenge so far was getting hospital leaders and CEOs on board. "If hospital leaders don't stand up and tell their doctors and nurses that patient safety is a priority then we've got some problems." It appeared to her that Duke and Hopkins were way ahead of other hospitals.

"When you're dealing with the health care industry," Karen said to me, "you're sometimes dealing with some pretty big egos. That's why it's so important for the doctors and nurses to hear your story. You come at it from a totally different perspective. They can't help but be moved and inspired by Josie's story. It's not necessarily that they don't *want* to change. It's just that they get so inundated with information all the time. They're busy, and they're being pulled in a million directions, and sometimes they just need to slow down, listen to the patient, and listen to each other. That's the message that you're so good at delivering."

Someone once told me that changing a culture can take years and years, and that it's one of the most difficult things to do. In a sense that was what people like Dr. Frush, Dr. Pronovost, and I were trying to do. We were trying to change the way doctors and nurses had been trained to think and act throughout their entire careers.

That evening there was a patient-safety reception to kick off the conference. Tables of food and a cocktail bar filled the middle of the large room, and twenty smaller tables lined the perimeter, each with displays on various patient-safety projects. Next to each display stood a nurse or two, proudly showcasing their patient-safety project. As I walked around the room talking to the nurses, I was amazed at what I saw. These projects ranged from decreasing hospital-acquired infections to improving teamwork. I wondered why practically everyone else was congregated around the food and wine tables. Why were they not looking at the projects that these nurses had worked so hard on and that could perhaps save a life?

On each display table sat a bowl of candy, and as I unwrapped a Hershey's Kiss and popped it into my mouth, I asked the nurse why there was so much candy. She confirmed what I had suspected: the candy was simply a lure to get people to look at the projects. I had seen this many times before at other patient-safety conferences: bowls of mints, Reese's Pieces, and M&M's beckoning people to walk over to the table, throw back some candy, and maybe glance at the project.

Sometimes, instead of candy I would see gimmicks or gifts, anything to make learning about patient safety *fun.* I cringed when I saw these things and when I saw people laughing as they browsed the displays. I wanted to stand on a table and wave my hands and say, *"Listen to me, listen to my story. Let me tell you why this is important!"* If I had a display it would be a handmade quilt with each square a picture of a patient who had died from medical errors. My quilt would cover the floor of this tremendous room. It would drape over the entire Cleveland Clinic.

As Karen and I walked together from one project to another, she explained some things that I didn't understand, like that a nosocomial infection was an infection acquired in the hospital. I asked her whether or not anybody would have come if there had not been food and wine.

She told me that they would have, and that I needed to understand that things like this didn't change overnight. "It's going to take baby steps. You and I both just need to keep doing what we do."

I looked at a group of doctors in the center of the room; they were laughing, sipping their wine, and eating ham biscuits. I thought of Jack at home, blowing out the candles on his birthday cake.

"I know. But I didn't come all this way for a cocktail party."

I sat in the first row in the amphitheater-like auditorium next to Karen. There were close to a hundred people in the audience and a hundred or so empty seats. I always wondered about the empty seats. Where were the others? Didn't they care? Peter Pronovost used to tell me that we just needed to cast a wider net. We have to hope that the people who hear us will go back and tell their coworkers.

I glanced at my notes as I listened to an executive welcome everyone and introduce me. He briefly described what had happened to Josie, then said, "And let us hope that by the grace of God this never happens to us at the Cleveland Clinic."

I sat there fixated on those words. Did he think that hope and God would prevent medical errors from occurring at his institution? If only it were as simple as that. It would take more than hope, much more, and placing the problem in someone else's hands was not going to work. He and his doctors and nurses needed to take ownership of the problem and fix it themselves.

The executive stepped down and shook my hand as I made my way to the stage. I walked up to the podium and watched him as he proceeded to climb the steps and then go out the door.

For a moment I was too stunned to speak. The room was silent, waiting for me to say something.

I looked at my notes and wondered why the executive had left the room, why he didn't want to hear what I had to say. I wanted to run after him and tell him that *he* was the one the audience needed to hear from. *He* was the one that needed to inspire the doctors and nurses to find ways to keep his hospital safe.

Frustrated and confused, I decided I didn't need my notes this time. I folded them up and put them in my pocket, not caring if I stumbled or messed up. I focused on the eyes of the doctors and nurses and began.

"Tonight is my son's eleventh birthday. I left him with the hope that I could inspire you tonight . . ."

I told Josie's story. I told the audience that simply hoping that medical errors would not happen to their institution was not going to prevent them. I told them what Peter Pronovost had told me so many times before and what Karen Frush and I had talked about earlier: "It's got to come from the top down. The leadership of each hospital must stand before their institution and tell their employees that patient safety is a priority."

I look back on that night and realize that the executive was probably just using the "grace of God" term as a figure of speech and that he didn't really mean it literally. Maybe he had an important meeting to go to when he walked out of the room, and perhaps I was being overly sensitive, but that night I couldn't let it go. I had to say something. I had sat on an airplane scared to death and I had left my son on his birthday. If I was going to continue to make sacrifices and work hard then so should the health care industry.

I had been to countless patient-safety conferences. I had seen patient-safety banners wave and buttons being worn. What happened after people heard me tell Josie's story? Was I someone who moved doctors and nurses just for that moment? Did they go back to their hospitals and carry on as they had before or was Josie's story actually changing their behavior? I was tired of making sacrifices; I wanted something in return. I wanted to be convinced that these hospitals meant what they were saying and I wanted to see it with my own eyes.

After that night I began asking each organization for information on exactly what they were doing to make care safer for their patients. I also asked them to tell me specifically why they wanted me to speak. Did they just need an inspirational orator or did they really and truly want to make their hospital safer?

The MHA, the Michigan Health and Hospital Association, a group consisting of all the hospitals in the state of Michigan, had established a goal to eliminate medical errors in all of the ICUs, intensive care units, in the state. It was a huge undertaking and would have to be done hospital by hospital, floor by floor. It could not be accomplished unless each doctor and each nurse from each ICU was 100 percent committed. The MHA could not force these hospitals to be a part of this mission; they had to convince them, and to do that they needed a face, a story, an inspiration. They used the Josie King story. One hundred and twenty-seven teams formed a coalition, a two-year program to be called the Keystone ICU project.

I didn't know exactly what the impact of Josie's story had been but I heard snippets about how the Keystone project was coming along. Two years later I was asked to come to Dearborn, Michigan, for the Keystone wrap-up. I could feel the emotion in the room as each hospital leader stood before the audience and shared the results. The Keystone project had been a huge success. It was estimated that 1,578 lives had been saved, patients spent 81,020 fewer days in the hospital, and hospitals saved over $165 million dollars because of the project. Before Keystone, Michigan was average in rankings of central-line infections. After Keystone, central-line infections in ICUs were reduced by nearly 50 percent. The Michigan Keystone Project would be covered in numerous medical journals and received extensive coverage in the national media.

I was proud to be sitting in the audience as the realization swept over me that this initiative had truly saved lives. I was proud of Chris Goeschel, the project leader whose fiery personality had kept these hospitals going over the two years. I was proud of Peter Pronovost, who had masterminded the project. But most of all I was proud of the hospitals that had chosen to come together two years ago, and that had worked hard to prevent medical errors.

I was startled when Chris Goeschel asked me to come up on stage. I made my way there and stood next to her. She opened a leather binder and read a letter:

Dear Tony and Sorrel,

"Keystone ICU" is our Michigan project to improve ICU care. As we approach the two-year anniversary of the partnership between John Hopkins Quality and Safety Research and the MHA Keystone Center, we are humbled by the dedication of the 127 teams we work with, and are in awe of their achievements.

Yet we know that work is just beginning, and the real challenges lie ahead. As we reflect on how we will lead these teams into uncharted waters and continue to push the envelope of what is possible, we are drawn to how it is that we have arrived at this place.

Josie's story is at the heart of our work with these teams. Yet the impact of the story transcends the tragic events that led to her death. In sharing the story, you demonstrate the best of what it is to be human and you challenge us to do the same. Emerson's words touch on what you have shown us: it is our capacity to tap what is deep within each of us that allows us to endure, to grow, and to make the world a better place.

The Michigan Keystone Project

She handed the book to me and I looked out into the audience as the applause turned into a standing ovation. I fought back tears, overcome with pride that Josie had been the inspiration for so much good.

In the cab to the airport I opened the brown leather binder. Inserted in each clear plastic sleeve was a personal letter from each ICU team leader, representing over thirty hospitals. Some of these letters were handwritten, some were typed.

. . . I am a nurse. I am testimony that Josie has a purpose bigger than any of us could have imagined. She has given life to many . . . Since the start of the project so much has progressed. We (nursing) actually have autonomy to call physicians on issues and concerns or questions of treatment plan . . . Thank you for giving us hope to communicate without worrying about hierarchy and "stepping on toes." . . . Thank you for the avoided complications and lives that have been saved . . .

From Holland Hospital

. . . Josie's story has catapulted a state, and I predict an industry, into action. At Gerber Memorial, the staff have become empowered to speak up, empowered to change, and empowered to make a difference for our patients. We've learned that it is okay to "rock the boat" if it means we will give the best care possible.

From Gerber Memorial Health Services

. . . You created a sense of urgency, and because of that, barriers were broken. We have made strides in improving the quality and safety of care for our patients; we have made more process improvements throughout our hospital in these past two years than we had in the previous ten years. The life and death of Josie is never far from our thoughts . . .

From Metro-Health Hospital

. . . Josie's story supplied us with the motivation to literally change the world, one patient at a time. Your loss has saved many others . . .

From St. Mary Mercy Hospital

. . . Thank you for having the courage to redirect your pain and suffering into an idea that has changed the culture in ICUs across the country. Staff have been empowered to give a voice to quality measurements that yield better outcomes as well as the delivery of more efficient care to their patients . . . You have given direction to staff and reawakened a passion for excellence . . . Josie will be remembered as a life that changed the practice of critical-care medicine in the world and you will be remembered as the mother that made that happen . . .

From Detroit Medical Center,
Huron Valley–Sinai Hospital

. . . Your experiences with health care have illuminated the fact that communication is paramount to ensuring patient safety. Some of our accomplishments: the elimination of ventilator-associated pneumonia, the elimination of bloodstream infections, increased senior executive awareness of unit-based safety concerns, better communication between staff, physicians, and families. Your commitment and Josie's story have galvanized a health care community into action.

From Detroit Medical Center,
Harper University Hospital

For the first time since I had begun this journey I was holding hard-core proof that Josie had indeed inspired positive change. Her life and death were making a difference.

I arrived home late that night and climbed into bed next to Tony, who blearily asked how my trip had been.

He rarely had time to get fully involved in the specifics of my work. Having bills to pay and mouths to feed, he didn't know the fine details of the organizations I was working with, the speeches I was making, or the programs that were being started. He only saw the big picture. That night I handed him the leather binder. I was glad that he could see, with his own eyes, evidence that we were making a difference—the three of us: Josie, Tony, and me.

18

As more and more people heard about what we had been through with Hopkins, they often remarked on how lucky we were. Even our friends who were doctors told us that we had gotten special treatment. I was confused and annoyed by these comments. Special treatment? It had not occurred to me that there was any other sort of treatment than what we had received. Obviously, I had thought, if a hospital makes a mistake, it will tell the family the truth, apologize, and fix the problem.

But because of the Josie King Web site and because of the *Good Morning America* exposure, I was beginning to hear from other people all around the country who had been affected by medical errors. They shared their stories with me and I began to realize that we had indeed been treated differently. We had received answers, we had been told that the problems would be fixed, and we had been apologized to. Many of these other people, however, had been stonewalled, turned away and shut down by the hospital.

Julie Koleszar had taken her two-year-old daughter, Charlotte, to the emergency room in Fallsbrook, California, at 4:30 p.m. after she had been vomiting throughout the day. As Julie sat in the waiting room, Charlotte continued to throw up. Julie tried to keep Charlotte hydrated, but the child could not keep the fluids down. Julie begged to be seen by a doctor. Finally, two hours later, they were admitted to an examination room, where they continued to wait for the doctor. Charlotte was becoming severely dehydrated. Julie begged the nurse to hook her daughter up to an IV but was turned down. Charlotte began throwing up blood and was having trouble breathing. Julie screamed for help as Charlotte's fingers and toes began turning blue. A doctor came in and inserted a breathing tube. Charlotte's heart rate plummeted. A trauma team was called and saw that the breathing tube had been inserted improperly. By this time, Charlotte's brain had been depleted of oxygen for too long and she was brain dead. Charlotte died later that night in her mother's arms.

The Koleszars wanted an explanation, they wanted answers, and they wanted an apology, but the hospital would not talk. They were forced to hire an attorney and, after two and a half years of a lengthy and costly lawsuit, the hospital offered a settlement and gave the family the answers they wanted. However, the Koleszars would never receive a sincere apology.

Dale Ann Micalizzi took her eleven-year-old son, Justin, to a hospital near their home in Albany, New York, to have fluid drained from his ankle from what appeared to be a sports injury. She kissed him as he was wheeled into the operating room and told him she'd see him soon. Justin never woke up. He died from complications.

Dale Ann and I became friends. We understood each other's anger and sadness. We talked often and sent each other cards on tough days like birthdays, anniversaries, and holidays. Our stories were similar but the paths we were on could not have been more different.

She knew Justin should not have died and that something had gone terribly wrong that day at the hospital. She asked questions, but no one gave her answers. She asked for his medical records and was given a box of jumbled, illegible documents.

Without any cooperation from the hospital, Dale Ann, like the Koleszars, was left with only one place to turn: the legal system. She tried to hire a lawyer to help her get answers but was repeatedly turned down, not because these lawyers didn't think the case could be won—it could. The reason was money.

Medical malpractice laws differ from state to state and in the year that Justin and Josie died, a jury could award a family upwards of one million dollars in states like Connecticut, Florida, and Texas, where there are no caps. These types of dollar figures make it very attractive for malpractice lawyers to take on these cases. However, in many states, including Maryland, there are caps on the amount a patient or a family can be awarded, with each state deciding what that amount should be. In New York at the time of Justin's death, there was a pecuniary loss rule, which was a special law pertaining to children: if a child dies of medical errors no award, or a severely limited award, would be granted. The reason: a child is of lesser economic value.

If Justin had been an adult, there would have been no cap and an attorney would have taken the case. Dale Ann would have gotten answers. With this pecuniary loss rule no lawyer could justify taking a case like Justin's. Even if they took on the case pro bono, they still needed to pay for medical experts and other expenses. No lawyer could afford to do it. Dale Ann gathered her life's savings and considered paying the attorneys hourly to take the case. They told her she would go bankrupt within a few months.

It didn't seem right that while I was working with hospitals and doctors to establish patient-safety programs and raise awareness, Dale Ann remained trapped in a lengthy legal battle, struggling simply to find out what had happened to her son.

"It keeps getting worse and worse," she would tell me. "I feel like I've been hit by a car, robbed, and then run over by the ambulance."

Dale Ann's and Julie's stories haunted me, as did many of the other stories that were quickly filling my in-box. I noticed that most of these stories had a common thread: the words, "The hospital didn't listen." These patients and families had no place to turn and, desperate for help and advice, they came to me, a person with no legal or medical background, their last resort. Feeling helpless, I often called upon Peter Pronovost, Rick Kidwell, or Paul Bekman to advise them. Other than listening and urging them to keep fighting, there was little I could do.

As I traveled around the country talking to hundreds and thousands of health care providers, I no longer wanted to tell just Josie's story. I wanted to tell them Justin's story and Charlotte's story. I wanted to stand up and tell them that theirs was a dysfunctional system.

Even as I was hearing from more and more families affected by medical errors, there were major health care industry players trying new, more transparent approaches in responding to unexpected events. UMHS, the University of Michigan

Health System, was looking into the reasons why some patients affected by medical errors ended up suing. They found that people tended to sue when they had unanswered questions and felt that they were not being told the truth.

In the year 2001, Richard Boothman, chief risk officer at UMHS, adopted a broad policy of engagement and disclosure. When there were questions about a patient's health, whether a mistake had been made or not, someone from within the hospital would go directly to the family, explain what had happened, and apologize if it was warranted. Claims began dropping in the very next year and have dropped every year since. After four years of this practice, the number of claims dropped by over half. The average time spent processing a malpractice claim went down to 9.5 months, from 20.3 months, and the system spent half as much on litigation costs. Richard Boothman was on to something. He had created a model that was what every patient deserved and was also saving his health system millions of dollars.

Not only was transparency making sense for patients and from a dollars perspective, it was also having clinical benefits. By encouraging doctors and nurses to report errors, performance improvement committees were able to review the errors and improve processes to prevent similar errors from happening again. Openness and disclosure were starting to look like the right thing to do from a variety of angles.

I got a call from Dr. Albert Wu, a medical researcher from Hopkins. Dr. Wu was doing a study on disclosure and transparency, more specifically, on the effects that lack of communication and lack of openness can have not only on the patients and family, but on the health care provider. We met in his office and he told me about the results of his study. He had concluded the same thing I had: most health care providers do not know how to treat a patient or a family when there has been an unexpected outcome, a mistake.

Telling a family, *your child died because we made a mistake* is painfully difficult, even for the most well intentioned. Sometimes it may seem less painful and easier to just retreat into the hospital and close off all communications with the family. Dr. Wu wanted to create a tool to help doctors and nurses realize the importance of opening the lines of communication, telling the family the truth, apologizing, and fixing the problem. He wanted to help create a tool to help them do the right thing. He asked if I would help and I agreed.

With his thorough Hopkins research, Josie's story, and my "from the patient's perspective" message, we created a program called "Removing Insult from Injury." It would consist of a DVD and a tool kit that would train doctors and nurses, along with other health care professionals, on how to treat a patient or family when a medical error has occurred.

19

I was becoming a recognizable face in the health care industry. Sometimes I felt like a poster child, a face for the statistics—a symbol of some sort. Somehow, I had stumbled upon this world, and for whatever reason, they had not only accepted me but invited me inside. In the beginning, I had felt awkward, out of place, and in way over my head. Eventually, though, I realized that I was no longer known as simply a mom on a mission. A new identity was being tacked to my name: national patient-safety advocate.

I had two completely separate lives. My life as a mother in Baltimore consisted of shuttling Jack, Relly, Eva, and Sam to and from school, soccer practice, tennis, lacrosse, and ski team, along with cooking, cleaning, and reading stories at night—trying hard to be a good mother.

And then there was my other life as a patient advocate. My parents, siblings, and friends had no idea what I was doing when I wasn't in a carpool line or on a lacrosse field and I didn't want to talk about my work. It was too hard to explain. It was between me and the health care industry.

In December of 2004, Dr. Berwick, the CEO of IHI, launched a tremendous campaign, the aim of which was to prevent a hundred thousand unnecessary deaths in the United States. Called the "100,000 Lives Campaign," the goal was to make this a national effort and achieve it in eighteen months. Dr. Berwick and IHI were challenging the entire health care industry—each and every hospital—to come together to prevent these needless deaths.

I had been asked by IHI to give a breakout session on disclosure at their annual conference in Orlando, Florida. Having been to this conference a few times over the years, I was amazed at how rapidly it was growing and how large it had become. The first IHI conference was held in 1989 with 287 attendees. Now, fifteen years later, in 2004, there would be representation from forty different countries and four thousand attendees on-site, with another ten thousand people watching via satellite. Judging by the sheer numbers it was apparent that the health care industry knew it had problems and wanted to fix them.

Dr. Berwick's star had steadily risen over the years. Extremely well liked and respected within the U.S. health care system, his influence was reaching abroad as well. The next year he would be knighted by the queen of England for his contributions to improving the British national health system. And throughout it all, he maintained a kind and humble demeanor while having the guts and courage to push thousands and thousands of health care providers toward goals that seemed impossible.

The hotel was buzzing with blue-shirted IHI staff racing around with walkie-talkies. One of them spotted me as I was checking in and told me that Don needed to see me immediately. I followed her through the crowd of people.

People I had gotten to know over the years waved and

said hello as we raced through the hotel. The sense of familiarity was comforting. We entered the conference room and spotted Don talking to a group of doctors and nurses. He was in his late fifties, with gray hair and a boyish grin.

He led me over to some chairs near the stage. We sat down and he explained to me that during his speech tomorrow some of the top leaders in the health care industry would be joining him on stage. He pointed to the seven chairs that were lined up next to the podium and rattled off the names: Dr. John Nelson, president of the American Medical Association; Barbara Blakeney, president of the ANA, the American Nurses Association; David Pryor, chief medical officer of Ascension Health; Dennis O'Leary, president of the Joint Commission; Dr. Jonathan Perlin, the undersecretary for health in the Department of Veterans Affairs; Dr. Steve Jencks, director of quality improvement at the Centers for Medicare and Medicaid Services; and Sister Mary Jean Ryan, president and CEO of SSM Health Care, one of the largest health care systems in the country.

I knew who these people were: they were important, the industry giants of American health care. These people, Don explained, would each be standing up after the campaign speech and addressing the audience. He then told me he had a favor to ask. Would I join the others on stage and address the audience?

I looked at the stage. I looked at the tremendous room, filled with thousands and thousands of chairs. The room was so immense that every two hundred feet a screen hung from above so that people could see the speaker without using binoculars.

I told him I had no idea what he would be talking about, I had nothing prepared, and I didn't belong up there.

"That's all right," he said, "just wing it. Speak from your heart. You're good at that, and you *do* belong up there."

There was electricity in the air the next morning as the blue shirts hustled about making last-minute preparations for the launch. Seats filled up well before the start and the press gathered. Huge banners that read "100,000 Lives" hung from the ceiling. I greeted my fellow panel members, some of whom I had met in previous years. I looked out at the sea of people, more people than I had ever seen in one room before in my life. We took our seats, mine at the end of the row.

Don began,

". . . I'm losing my patience. Maybe it's my age. Maybe it's the e-mails from people who keep telling me what went wrong with their care . . .

"So, here's what I think we should do. I think we should save one hundred thousand lives. And I think we should do that by June 14, 2006—eighteen months from today. Some is not a number; soon is not a time. Here's the number: one hundred thousand. Here's the time: June 14, 2006—9 a.m.

. . . The theme for this campaign is "How?" It comes directly from a poignant e-mail I got last year from a doctor who wrote basically this: "I get it. I get it. I get it. You don't have to tell me one more time how bad health care quality is, or how much better we can be. You don't have to tell me one more time *what* to accomplish. I know what. What I need now is the *how*."

I looked out at the riveted audience while Don explained the *hows*.

"The following interventions will be the route to success. I am going to ask that we get these six changes, these interventions—all of them—into sixteen hundred American hospitals within the next year."

He began listing the six changes.
1. Reliable, evidence-based care for acute myocardial infarctions (heart attacks).
2. Use of the so-called ventilator bundle, a set of scientifically validated processes used for management of ventilated patients to help prevent ventilator-acquired pneumonia.
3. Use of the central line bundle to keep in-dwelling central venous catheters from becoming infected.
4. Prevention of surgical site infections, largely by reliable use of appropriately chosen and appropriately timed peri-operative antibiotic.
5. Prevention of severe adverse drug events, largely through the use of so-called medication reconciliation procedures.

Some of it was over my nonclinical head, but most of it made sense to me. His final intervention was something called rapid response teams. I had heard the term over the years but knew very little about it.

"Rapid response teams. Hospitals create these teams to respond immediately to clinicians—usually nurses—who are getting worried about a patient, often only a gut feeling. Something can be going wrong with Mrs. Smith, even if he or she can't put his or her finger on it. In the usual system, these worries can lie there, unresolved, not responded to, for a long time—a day or two, or more. Meanwhile, too often, Mrs. Smith slips into worse and worse shape, sort of under our noses. An urgent clinical response finally happens only when disaster strikes—when her heart stops and a code blue is called."

I listened to his every word, realizing that what happened to Mrs. Smith was exactly what happened to Josie.

"Rapid response teams come sooner. They come to Mrs. Smith's bedside when someone gets worried. A nurse or other clinician can call them on his or her own initiative and the team comes right away. They assess the patient urgently, form an impression, and make a plan. They're trying to prevent the disaster that might have occurred later on—hours or days later. Often they do."

I relived Josie's death like a high-speed slide show, and I realized this was the answer. A rapid response team would have saved her.

I could not concentrate on the rest of Don's speech. My mind was reeling. Yes, yes, yes. *This* was the solution. *This* was it. As each of the executives stood up, endorsed the campaign, and pledged their support, I was in another world.

I was at the hospital with Josie. *I* pushed the button. *I* called the rapid response team. They came. Josie lived.

The microphone was handed to me as Don introduced me to the audience.

I had no idea what to say or where to start. I looked out into the huge audience and decided to do what Don had told me: wing it, speak from the heart. I brought the microphone in close and I told the audience that the campaign made me feel both happy and sad. "I'm happy because I know it will save lives. I'm sad because I wish it had been in place a few years ago when Josie was in the hospital." I told them how excited I was about rapid response teams, a team of fresh eyes to evaluate the patient.

I paused, not sure if I should ask the question that was racing through my mind, not sure if I had the courage to suggest something that I knew would seem absurd to many in the audience. I decided that I didn't care if I made a complete fool of myself. I didn't care if they laughed at me, I had to ask.

"Do you think a patient or family member could push the button? Could they call the rapid response team to the bedside if no one was listening to them and they were scared out of their minds?"

I knew that the thought of giving a patient or a family this sort of power was pretty much unheard of in the health care industry. But as I stood there, something strange happened in the audience. There were sighs and then slow clapping. The clapping spread as some people began to rise from their seats. I continued, "I believe with all of my heart that if I had been able to call a rapid response team, my daughter Josie would not have died. She would be six years old, and I wouldn't be standing here today."

The room went silent as I handed the microphone back to Don.

That afternoon, I stood at the same podium with a fraction of the former audience, perhaps a few hundred. The speaker before me was Linda Kenney and she shared the stage with Dr. Rick van Pelt. Theirs was a fascinating story and demonstrated one of the shortcomings of our health care system. Linda was admitted to Brigham and Women's Hospital in Boston to undergo ankle replacement surgery. Dr. van Pelt, her anesthesiologist, began administering the drug to numb her lower leg. Minutes later, she had a grand mal seizure followed by cardiac arrest. After hours of open-heart surgery, the cardiac emergency team was able to stabilize her. When Linda woke up, instead of a mended foot she had a fourteen-inch scar that ran from the bottom of her neck to her abdomen. The doctors told her that she had suffered an allergic reaction to the anesthesia.

Dr. van Pelt could not sleep for days. He knew that Mrs. Kenney was not allergic to the drugs: he had mistakenly administered the drug to her circulatory system instead of her nervous system.

He wanted to talk to her. He wanted to apologize, but the hospital told him to not contact her. Weeks later, fully aware that he was defying the hospital and would most likely lose his job, he wrote Linda an apology letter. They talked on the phone and, six months later, Linda founded an organization called MITSS, Medically Induced Trauma Support Services, with the help and support of Dr. van Pelt. Their mission was "To Support Healing and Restore Hope" to patients, families, and clinicians after a medically-induced trauma.

The audience could not help but be moved by these two, especially young Dr. van Pelt, who demonstrated to the doctors, nurses, and administrators what it is to be human: that is, to make a mistake and to want to fix it. The right way. I was glad they had the courage to stand up and share their story.

I looked at my watch and realized that Rick and Linda had unknowingly gone over their allotted time, leaving me with less than ten minutes. I decided that instead of talking about patient safety or disclosure, I would tell the audience about the e-mails I had received from patients and families who had been affected by medical errors.

"They write to me because they have nowhere else to go," I told them. "They're desperate to find answers, but what can I do? I'm not a doctor or a lawyer. I'm not an expert on any of this. I can only listen to them. I need your help."

I asked the audience, each doctor and nurse, to write their name, phone number, and hospital on a piece of paper. "That way, when a patient comes to me, I can look through the slips of paper for a match. If there is one, I can call on you and perhaps, together, we can help that patient, that family."

At the end of the session, I stood by the door like a beggar with my hands cupped as people handed me slips of paper, business cards, and letters. I couldn't hold all of the scraps, so I laid them on the table and watched the pile grow bigger and bigger. After everyone had left the room, I quickly shuffled through the little slips, hoping that I would come across the name of the hospital in Albany where Dale Ann's son had died. I didn't find it.

A year later, I was once again back at the annual IHI conference. This time Dale Ann was there. She and I had continued to communicate often over the years. We made a good team, trying together to help the many families who had contacted us.

She looked tired when I saw her standing alone near the Christmas tree. We sat down on a couch in the middle of the large hotel lobby, two mothers whose lives had been derailed by the health care industry, two outsiders surrounded by a sea of doctors, nurses, and administrators. I asked her what the latest was with her case and she told me that Don Berwick had contacted the hospital in Albany to try to mediate, but nothing had yet transpired.

"They never apologized or admitted anything," she told me.

Don had been her only hope. It had been five years and her statute of limitations was up. There was nothing else she could do.

I wanted to tell her to keep fighting, but the truth was, she was fighting a losing battle. So I told her something that so many people had said to me, something that had made me cringe every time I heard it. I hated myself for saying it. I told her to move on.

We continued talking and I tried to be positive and help her look on the bright side, but there wasn't one.

The next morning Dale Ann and I sat next to each other in the same room where Don had launched the "100,000 Lives" campaign a year ago. Again there were thousands of people in attendance. Don shared with the audience Justin's tragic story. He spoke of Dale Ann's long hard fight. Dale Ann had tears in her eyes. I put my hand out and she held on to it.

* * *

"Dale Ann," Don said, "I apologize. I so wish I could apologize to Justin himself, but that chance is lost. We can apologize to Dale Ann, though," he said to the audience. "We can say we are sorry. It happened on our watch. No one in this room, I suspect, actually took care of Justin directly, but I believe that we can, and should, accept collective responsibility for not yet having built a health care world safe enough for him, and for tens of thousands of patients and families who are injured in our care. Dale Ann, I am so so sorry."

He asked the audience to stand for a moment of silence, a symbol of the health care industry's apology to Dale Ann. As I stood up to join the rest of the audience, Dale Ann would not let go of my hand. I sat with her as the audience stood silently all around us. I looked up at Don. His head was bowed and his shoulders were slumped. Doctors, nurses, CEOs, and administrators—thousands of them—were standing in silence, thinking of Justin, standing in silence out of respect, regret, and sadness for his mother, offering her the one thing she had been searching for for so many years, an apology, a sincere apology.

It became clearer to me that day that we all wanted a safer health care system. Not just people like me and Dale Ann, but doctors, nurses, and CEOs. Everyone. American health care *was* going to be safer. We were going to do it, together. We were going to turn the battleship around through patient-safety programs, through new technology, through a new culture, and through stories like Josie's and Justin's.

* * *

It was 9 p.m. when I finally got home. I thanked Ron, the driver, and walked toward the back door as the dogs ran up to greet me. I took my shoes off and tiptoed up the stairs. Putting my bag down, I peeked in and saw the children lying in our bed with Tony. Jack, Relly, and Eva were reading to themselves while Tony read *The Berenstain Bears* to Sam, who was falling asleep.

"Mom's home," Eva said, when she spotted me.

I blew her a kiss and leaned over to pick Sam up. He was wearing his blue race-car pajamas and he wrapped his arms around my neck and laid his head on my shoulder as I carried him into his room. I breathed in the sweet smell of his just-washed hair and laid him down on his bed. I went back and sat with Tony and the other kids.

I was always coming home with little knickknacks from the conferences: pens, pencils, bags, notepads, coffee mugs. Sometimes the hospitals gave me beautiful, meaningful gifts: coffee table books about the hospital, pewter cups, leather binders. Knowing I hated leaving my children, they often sent me home with stuffed animals and little gifts for each of them. Other times they gave me plaques with inscriptions thanking me for helping them. The most special gift I ever received was a quilt handmade by a group of nurses from Abington, Pennsylvania.

This time, I reached into my heavy red briefcase and threw them each a mini hand sanitizer, a lanyard with a pen attached, a key chain, and a red, white, and blue patient-safety button.

They rifled through their treats, squeezed the hand sanitizer into their hands, and pinned their patient-safety buttons on their bathrobes as they told me about their day.

I listened to them rattle on about all the great things they had done with their father and it was pretty clear to me that the separation was much harder on me than it was on them.

As Tony and I tucked the children into bed he asked me how the trip had been. I told him it was great.

"Are you glad you went?"

"Yeah, I'm really glad I went." And I realized that as much as I hated public speaking, hated the airplanes, and hated leaving my family I was always glad I went.

We went downstairs to turn off the lights and lock the doors. The little twinkly Christmas tree lights cast a warm glow throughout the old living room. As I bent down to unplug them, Tony said, "Let's just sit here for a minute and look at the tree."

As the two of us sat on the sofa looking at the Christmas tree I realized that something felt different. I didn't feel the horrible dread of the holidays that I had felt those first few years after Josie had died. I was actually looking forward to Christmas, being with friends and family, the holiday parties, the cooking, the presents, the commotion.

"Does this Christmas feel different to you?" I asked, as I put my feet on the coffee table.

"Yeah, it does," he answered. "I think this will be the best Christmas we've had in a long time."

He stood up to check the water level in the tree stand.

"Do you think it's because of time passing? Do you think that's what makes it easier?"

"I think it's time, and I think we've learned how to live without her," he said.

He sat back down next to me. "You know, I think we should have a party, a big Christmas party."

Torches lined the driveway that Christmas, fires were lit in every fireplace, Christmas music wafted throughout the house, the lights were dimmed and candles flickered in every room, and the children passed hors d'oeuvres and ham biscuits. The old house had become our home again. It was filled with family and friends, and there was laughter.

20

I received a call from Tami Merryman, who had been spear-heading innovative safety programs at the University of Pittsburgh Medical Center for several years. Tami told me she had been in the audience that day in Orlando when I posed the question of whether a patient or family member could call a rapid response team. She told me that they were going to do it—they were going to create a patient/family-activated rapid response team at UPMC Shadyside Hospital. I was surprised that someone in the audience was actually going to follow through with allowing patients and their families such access. I knew it was more than a bold move. I imagined that to some it was unheard of. Tami said it would be called "Condition Help" or the "Josie King Call Line." She asked if I would be involved and I accepted.

Their plan was to set up an internal phone number that patients or their families could call from the bedside if they felt they were experiencing or saw a serious change in patient condition that was not getting sufficient attention from the floor staff. A hospital operator, who would be trained on how to field the calls, would listen to the concerns and then alert the rapid response team, which would consist of doctors, nurses, and a patient-relations coordinator. They would evaluate the patient and develop a plan for care.

Tami also developed an impressive series of material to help the staff respond to issues, record information, and evaluate the outcomes.

As I spent time with Tami and her team, various issues arose. One was an issue that most of the health care establishment had, concerning the notion of involving patients and families: how to prevent patients or families from abusing the system, calling when the food tastes bad, or when they dropped the remote control.

We decided that the best way to prevent unwarranted calls was to educate the patient and family. This would be done in a number of ways, one of which was through creating educational brochures that would explain to the patient and family what Condition Help was, when to call it, and when not to call it. To make this brochure have more of an impact, we decided that a picture of Josie should be placed on the front. Patients would realize that Condition Help was put in place to prevent others from being harmed or killed like this little girl. How could they abuse a system like that?

Another issue that arose was how to get skeptical physicians and other staff members on board. As always, this came down to leadership. Tami was an energetic and persuasive leader who had a keen sense of humor and was passionate about patient safety. As I became more and more involved in the health care industry, I was beginning to realize that I had seen these very same qualities in practically all of the patient-safety leaders I had met. Tami stood in front of a room full of skeptics and asked them to consider offering Condition Help to the Shadyside patients because, as she said, "it's the right thing to do." She used Josie's story and quickly had them convinced.

A few months later Shadyside Hospital launched Condition Help. The pilot proved to be a success. It was well liked by hospital staff and patients and their families.

Not long after Shadyside implemented Condition Help the Children's Hospital of Pittsburgh, another UPMC affiliate, decided to do the same. With some initial funding from the Josie King Foundation they were up and running within a few months. It felt good to know that patients like Josie and parents like me now had a great resource available to them, a resource that could potentially save a life.

Eighteen months after Shadyside's initial pilot and a year after the Children's Hospital, Tami decided to bring together the twelve other UPMC hospitals with the hope that perhaps they, too, would want to implement the program. She asked me if I would kick off the event with a speech. I flew up the night before and had dinner with Tami and a number of Condition Help leaders. I asked one of the nurse leaders how things were going at her unit. She told me it was all great, but they had not had the big event. I asked her what she meant. "You know the we-saved-a-life big event." That night I thought about what she had said and I wondered about the big event.

The next morning, I stood behind the podium and talked about all of the reasons I believed in Condition Help. As I got ready to step down from the podium I decided to say something about the big event.

"Who cares about the big event? There may never *be* a big event. If I had been able to call for help," I said, "the team would have come, they would have looked at Josie, and they would have said, 'Patient is thirsty. Give her water.'

206

There would not have been a big event. Josie would have gotten fluids and she would be alive."

While I stood there, I decided to bring up another issue that had always confused me. I had come to learn that the health care industry places tremendous value on scientific data. Everything had to be measured, and backed up by facts, figures, and data. There had been questions raised as to how Condition Help could be measured, how scientific data could be collected.

I told the audience that I understood the importance of scientific data and I respected the need for it. "I can imagine that a program like Condition H must be a hard thing to quantify or document. How do you measure lives *potentially* saved? But can't this be done just because it's the right thing to do? Can't it be done because patients and families might feel more comfortable, and actually *privileged* to be given this opportunity? Can't it be done because maybe, just maybe, it might change the culture? Don't you think that the next time a mother says to one of your doctors or nurses, 'something isn't right, can you come look,' that they will slow down and take a good look because they know that otherwise, that mother will call a rapid response team." I told the audience that I could not make a business case for Condition Help. I didn't know if its success could be measured and scientific data published in medical journals. I couldn't promise them that their patients wouldn't abuse it.

There was only one thing I could say with certainty. "Look deep within your organization and at least consider giving your families and patients this privilege, this right. If you think it's a good idea, then find a way to make it work. In doing this, I believe you will save lives."

*   *   *

Condition Help has become known throughout the nation, with hospitals coming to the Josie King Foundation and to UPMC wanting to learn more so that they, too, can find a way to implement a family-activated rapid response team. And we actually do have some data. UPMC reported that 90 percent of patients who called Condition Help would call it again if they felt it was needed, 100 percent of callers felt their needs were met by the team, and 69 percent of the calls revealed that potentially harmful patient situations would have occurred if Condition Help had not been called. For many, the doubts about giving patients and their families such access have been erased. But beyond the data, many hospitals are implementing Condition Help because they believe it is simply the right thing to do.

I was excited about Condition Help and the impact it could have not only on patients but on the culture of the health care industry, and as I spoke to a friend of mine one day it dawned on me that there might be another little way in which the Josie King Foundation could not only help patients but, again, help change the culture. My friend's father had suffered a stroke and was in the hospital. She asked me what she should do to make sure he got the best treatment possible.

I told her to pay attention and write everything down and I handed her a small spiral notebook. The next morning, as I was running in the woods, I thought about my friend and wondered if she was using the notebook I had given her. I thought back to when Josie had been at the hospital and how writing had helped me stay organized and gave me a sense of control. And then it hit me—the Josie King Foundation needed to create a journal specifically for patients and families.

I sprinted home, sat at my desk, and began sketching out ideas. The journal had to be small enough to fit into a pocket-book or briefcase; it had to have thirty days' worth of pages; each day—each page—needed to have prompts, suggesting what to keep track of. I ran upstairs to the attic and rummaged through condolence letters and medical records until I found my journal. I looked at all of the different things I had kept track of: parking space number, medical team on duty, daily goals, medications, surgery, procedures, questions to ask. These, I decided, would be the prompts.

I called it the Care Journal. The cover would be green, the color of hope, with a small leaf, the symbol of the Josie King Foundation, in the center.

I took a prototype of the little green journal with me to my next speaking engagement. I sat at the dinner table with a group of nurses and told them my idea as I proudly passed the Care Journal around the table.

"Isn't it great? Look how pretty it is. Look how useful it is. Your patients are going to love it," I said excitedly, but all they did was look at the book, look at each other, and then look at me. They told me that sometimes when doctors and nurses see someone sitting in the corner writing it makes them feel uncomfortable. "They feel like they're being documented. They see it as a potential lawsuit," one of the nurses said.

"They call them scribblers," another nurse added.

I was confused by their response. Lawsuits? It made no sense to me. I asked them what they did when their father or their child was in the hospital.

"We document everything. We write it all down."

And so we talked and we brainstormed.

We all agreed that there was a disconnect, a feeling of mistrust between health care providers and patients. If the Care Journal came from the hospital, not from me or the Josie King Foundation, perhaps we could help bridge the disconnect.

I popped a sample in the mail to the health care editor at the *Wall Street Journal*. A week later they ran an article about it, and e-mails from patients and families, hospitals, and large health care systems began to flood my in-box. The next day, I called the printer in Pennsylvania and told them to start the presses. I needed ten thousand Care Journals.

Within months, over a dozen hospitals had partnered with the Josie King Foundation to get Care Journals into the hands of their patients. Inserted in many was a note from the hospital to the patient that read:

> Welcome to our hospital. We value our patients, your family, and the feedback you provide us. Please accept this Care Journal as a gift. We hope you use this as a place to keep track of information and questions as they may arise. We encourage you to partner with us in your care.

Thousands of Care Journals are being used by patients all over the country. I'd like to think that perhaps it is more than just a little green book. I'd like to think that perhaps, like the Condition Help program, it is helping to change the culture by bridging the disconnect that is so often felt between patients and their families and the health care provider.

21

I was on my way out the door to pick the children up from school when the phone rang. The caller's name was Dr. Mike Finley. He told me he was a doctor at CHRISTUS St. Michael Health System in Texarkana, Texas, and he asked if I would come to St. Michael in the spring. I told him that I was cutting back on speaking engagements and Texas was just too far. I was throwing snacks in my bag and looking for my keys when something he said caught my attention.

"I can get a room full of nurses to come to a talk about patient safety, but I can't seem to get one physician to listen to me," he said. "I've tried everything."

My mind flashed back to all of the audiences that I had stood before and all of the health care providers that I had met since Josie's death. The more I thought about it, the more it dawned on me: it was the nurses who seemed to dominate the audiences, it was the nurses who seemed to initiate patient-safety programs, and it was the nurses who seemed to be more eager to make systems safer. I thought about how I had heard, over and over again, nurses' desire for better communication between themselves and doctors. Where were all the doctors? Were they too busy? Did they think that this was not their problem? I decided I would be five minutes late for carpool and would listen to what else Dr. Finley had to say.

He told me he saw medical errors and near misses happening too often. "Most of the time it's because doctors and nurses just aren't working well together. It always seems to come down to a breakdown in communication."

"What exactly do you think I can do?" I asked.

He wanted me talk to the physicians. "If you can help me convince one physician to be a part of the movement, it'll make a difference."

I knew there would not be a direct flight to Texarkana and that I would have to spend the night, but I believed in what Dr. Finley was fighting for. It was February, and May was months away, so I agreed to do it.

I put Dr. Finley in touch with my brother-in-law Jay and they talked about the Patient Safety Group initiative. By this time, the Patient Safety Group was three years old and had made great strides. eCUSP, Peter Pronovost's patient safety tool that we had made electronic, was now in nearly fifty hospitals and long-term health care facilities, including some of the top pediatric hospitals in the country. Dr. Finley asked Jay to come along, meet the team from St. Michael, and talk to them about the patient-safety tool.

Texarkana is a small, country town and the Texas-Arkansas state line runs smack down the middle of it and through the small post office building. The town is made up largely of blue-collar laborers, most of whom work in the paper mills and farm equipment factories. Those who don't are teachers, lawyers, or employees at St. Michael, a small multipurpose acute-care hospital.

At the tiny Texarkana airport, Jay and I were greeted by

a number of St. Michael's administrators and an over-the-top-friendly man named Jeffrey, who told us he would be driving us to the hotel. Jeffrey explained our itinerary for the next twenty-four hours. Dr. Finley and his wife would be picking us up at the hotel at 6:30 and would drive us and the other speaker, a physician by the name of Dr. Red Duke, to Park Place, a favorite local restaurant.

I didn't know anything about Dr. Duke, or that we were even presenting together. I had never presented with a doctor other than Dr. Pronovost, but perhaps having a doctor with me, sending the same message, would make it easier to sway the doctors in the audience.

We loaded our bags into the back of Jeffrey's white Chevrolet while he, in great detail, explained the reason for his limp, which neither Jay nor I had noticed. He told us he had been walking in his backyard and fell into a window well. "I was hollerin' and hollerin' for my girlfriend, but she was watching TV and couldn't hear me," he said. "Finally, after an hour, she heard me and sent down a ladder."

I wondered how someone could walk right into a window well. I quickly hopped into the back seat and Jay gave me a shove with his elbow as he slid up front next to Jeffrey.

As we drove down the road toward the hotel, we listened as Jeffrey explained why houses in Texas don't have basements. "The land's just too darn soft," he told us, "and we're below sea level, so when it rains there's an awful lot of moodoo that builds up."

"Moodoo?" I asked.

"You know, moodoo, the green bacteria stuff that grows when there's a lot of moisture in the air." Oh yes, *mildew,* I thought, realizing I needed to tune my ear to his thick accent.

Somewhere in the midst of hearing about the moodoo in Texas and the falling-in-the-hole episode, he asked us if we would like a tour of Texarkana. Before we had a chance to respond, the white Chevy was turning around and on its way into the heart of town.

I rolled down the window and wondered how Relly had done on her geography test and if Sam had enjoyed his first day of soccer. Tony was probably making quesadillas for dinner. Jeffrey drove us back and forth across the Texas-Arkansas state line, demonstrating how Texarkana had gotten its name. He showed us where Ross Perot had grown up and where Scott Joplin had taken music lessons. Somehow, though, Jeffrey got the picture that maybe we should get back to the hotel and check in before Dr. Finley picked us up. On the way back, he said he had to show us just one more thing, the all-time best restaurant in town. He slowed the white Chevy down and pointed to Bryce's Cafeteria. He told us they served "the best homemade peach pie in all of Texas."

When we arrived at the hotel—the Comfort Inn on the outskirts of town—Jay and I thanked him, said good-bye, and hightailed it to our rooms to get ready for dinner. Back downstairs we sat outside, waiting for Dr. Finley to pick us up. It was a warm night and as the sun began to set the neon lights popped on in the strip mall across the highway. It felt good to be outside and to feel the warm Texas air. In the parking lot, a man with a cowboy hat was cussing as he struggled to remove a suitcase from the back of a pickup truck. As he walked toward us, still muttering angrily, I took in his scruffy mustache, his faded Levi's that were a smidge too tight, and his motorcycle jacket. He looked to be in his sixties and was worn and weathered and handsome in an odd sort of way. He was the real-deal Texas cowboy and I suspected he was in town for a local rodeo. As he got closer, I made out the name that was stitched on his jacket: Red Duke, MD.

"Well, you must be Sorrel King. I recognize you from your DVD," he said. "I'm Red Duke. It sure is nice to meet you, sweetie."

This was not what I had been expecting. Not at all. There was no way this guy could be a surgeon. Maybe a cowboy-farmer or a cowboy-builder, or even a cowboy-teacher, but there was surely no such thing as a cowboy-surgeon. I shook his hand and wondered how this was going to play out.

Dr. Finley and his wife Nancy arrived to drive Jay and me to Park Place. Dr. Duke would meet us there. As we drove to the restaurant, Nancy told us how much she appreciated us coming to Texarkana. "I hope you don't mind if a few people join us for dinner," Dr. Finley said. "Everyone has been so inspired by your story and your work. We just couldn't turn them down."

Red and I were seated at one end of the table, and fifteen or so doctors, nurses, and administrators filled the rest of the chairs. Chris Karam, the St. Michael's CEO, and his wife Michelle, sat across from me. Chris had just been appointed CEO of St. Michael's a year earlier, although he looked to be no more than thirty-five. In spite of his youth, he seemed like a nice, smart guy who was well respected. Michelle, pretty with a southern accent, leaned across the table and whispered in my ear.

"I want you to know that I have been following Josie's story and your work, and I believe God is with you every single step of the way." She told me she was glad that I had come to St. Michael to share Josie's story. "I think it'll make a difference," she said.

It was nice to know that Josie was reaching beyond nurses and doctors to the wives of CEOs. My mother always said that behind every successful man is a successful woman, and Michelle seemed like just the kind of woman who would make sure her CEO husband followed through on his promises to make his hospital safer.

At the far end of the table was a nun, a real nun, habit and all. Her name was Sister Damian, and she was from Cork, Ireland. She was soft-spoken but I could tell she commanded respect. Those around her hung on her every word.

After Red arrived we ordered drinks. Then he asked if he could escort me to the salad bar and insisted on holding my plate for me as I piled on the beets and croutons. I told him it was really not necessary and that I truly was able to hold my own plate.

"Darlin', you just let me take care of things. You sit yourself on down," he said. As we ate our salad he told me about the trauma unit he had started at Memorial Hermann in Houston and his life as a surgeon in Afghanistan. The vision of this cowboy-surgeon in Afghanistan added to his mystique.

We ordered dessert and coffee, and as Red got into a heated conversation with Chris, the CEO, about college football, I snuck down to visit Sister Damian at the other end of the table. There wasn't a chair, so I knelt next to her. She held my hands in hers and in a thick Irish accent told me that she was proud of what I was doing. She then closed her eyes and started to pray. I told her, as she continued to hold my hands in hers, that I was not much of a religious person. "I wish I was. I've tried, but I just couldn't figure it out." I told her that the first time I ever thought there could possibly be a God was the day I learned Josie was going to die. "What happened to Josie was so unbelievable that I knew it had to be God," I told her.

She looked at me and was quiet for a moment before she spoke. "My dear, it was not God who took Josie," she told me. "It was mankind. God is at work now using you and Josie to send a message."

I had never thought of it like that. God didn't want Josie to die but he was using her to deliver a message? It sort of made sense. Sister Damian continued whispering her prayers as she leaned in close to me. I was glad to be kneeling on the floor where no one could see me.

That night I lay in bed thinking about Sister Damian. All along I had been thinking that God had planned this: the water heater, the accident, her thirst, the methadone, no one listening, the compounded errors. What Sister Damian had said was making more sense: God didn't want Josie to die. Her death was human error, a result of mankind's flaws. Sister Damian's words rang in my head, "Now God is using you and Josie to send a message."

Maybe she was right. I figured she had to know what she was talking about: she had dedicated her whole life to figuring out this type of stuff. Perhaps there was a God—not because Josie died but, as Sister Damian had said, because I had survived. Maybe I didn't feel God speaking to me, didn't understand the hymns and prayers, didn't understand the purpose of going to church, but it was becoming clear to me that somehow I had found the strength and courage to do things I never thought I could.

217

*   *   *

Early the next morning I sat in the dining room waiting for Red to join me for breakfast. He walked in wearing a suit and his cowboy hat and I could immediately tell he felt uncomfortable in the suit. He said good morning, calling me "darlin'" as he leaned over me, and plopped his cowboy hat on the seat across from me. He asked if I'd order him some fried eggs, over easy, and black coffee, and told me he'd be right back. As I watched him walk across the dining room I noticed that everyone else was also watching him. A man came up to me with a camera in his hand and asked if that was Red Duke I was with. I told him it was and asked if he was famous or something.

"Hell, yeah, he's a big deal. Where are you from?"

"Baltimore," I said, feeling somewhat embarrassed.

"Well, Red Duke's famous, at least to anyone in Texas. He is a big damn deal."

I wasn't going to ask why, for fear of looking like even more of an idiot.

When Red came back to the table the man asked him for his autograph and if he could take a picture. As the man's wife took photos of the two, I wondered if Red had ever spent this much time with someone who had absolutely no idea who he was. He sat down with a sheepish look on his face. I watched as he ate his eggs and asked him just exactly who he was.

"Honey, I ain't nothin' but an old country doc," he said. "How 'bout you pass me that there salt."

I had never been called honey or darlin' so many times before, and I was beginning to like it. I looked around the room. All eyes were glued on us. I passed him the salt.

Jay met us after breakfast and we were all picked up by Dr. Finley and taken to St. Michael. We arrived at the hospital, where it became clear just how big of a deal Dr. Red Duke was. Nurses and doctors surrounded him and shook his hand. Pictures were taken. Chris, the CEO, whisked him off to meet some of the local politicians as Jay and I were led to a room full of nurses.

St. Michael, a fairly new hospital, had big windows that opened up on to beautiful gardens and walking paths, giving it a warm and sunny feel. Jay and I followed Dr. Finley down the freshly carpeted halls that led to the conference room and I heard a voice come over the loudspeaker. It was Sister Damian, praying for the patients, the doctors, and the nurses.

Six months prior to my coming to Texarkana, Dr. Finley had asked thirty nurses to give him an hour of their time before they began their morning shift, promising them a breakfast buffet. The best way to get a group of people to come to an early meeting, he had told me, was to offer food, good food. It worked. He popped in the *Josie King Story* DVD and turned off the lights. The nurses put down their forks and listened to Josie's story unfold. When he flicked the lights back on and walked to the podium, he saw some of them wipe away tears. The room had been silent as Dr. Finley spoke of errors and near misses that were occurring not only in hospitals in Texas but all around the country.

"We owe it to our patients, we owe it to ourselves, and we owe it to this little girl to do something."

He shared with them a game plan and asked if anyone would like to be a part of it. All thirty nurses raised their hands.

Now, six months later, Jay and I were sitting in on their biweekly meeting and they shared with us all of the patient-safety initiatives that were under way. I listened to each team leader address the group about the specific project they had been working on since seeing Josie's story.

At the end of their presentations, Dr. Finley introduced me and asked if I had any thoughts I'd like to share. I stood up and thanked the nurses for all of their hard work. I told them how much it meant to be able to see firsthand that Josie's story had inspired such amazing patient-safety projects. "Before I introduce Jay King there is one thing I need to clarify," I said. "Jay is *not* my husband." I told them that everywhere we went, people thought we were married. "I actually married his much younger, more handsome, brother," I said.

From across the room a nurse yelled out, "Sweetheart, if I had a husband half as handsome as Jay, I sure wouldn't be leaving him at home." Everyone laughed and craned their necks to take a look at Jay, who was turning bright red.

After the meeting, one of the nurses asked if I'd like a tour of the hospital. I had been on many hospital tours and was always amazed by what I saw, and considered it a privilege to witness doctors and nurses at work. As we rode the escalator up to the second floor she said to me, "The most important part of St. Michael's rides up and down this escalator every day—the employees, the doctors, and nurses."

She asked if she could take me to the fourth floor. There was a nurse whose four-year-old son had recently been killed in a car accident. "Her name is Tammy," she said. "She'd like to meet you."

Over the years, since Josie had died, I had become sort of a go-to girl for people who had suffered a loss. Sometimes people would share their stories with me about their beloved grandmother who had passed away or about an aunt or uncle or perhaps a parent. Most of the time I would kindly tell that person that I really couldn't help them because I did not know what losing a grandmother or an aunt or uncle felt like. And privately, although I felt guilty for feeling this way, I believed my loss was greater than theirs. There is no loss in life greater than losing a child.

However, when someone tells me about a mother whose child has just died, I will drop everything and run to her as fast as I can. I will put my arms around her and let her cry on my shoulder. I will pull her hair back from her tear-streaked face and look into her lost eyes and tell her I understand.

Sadly, over the years, I have faced too many of these mothers who have lost children. My friend Beth's daughter drowned in the summer of 2003. Lynn's three-year-old daughter died in a construction accident in 2004. Susan's sixteen-year-old son died in a car accident in the spring of 2004. Laura's eight-year-old daughter died of a rare illness in March of 2007. I offered my phone numbers to those who I did not know well, and they called me. They talked, and I listened. Often, I took my brown box of grief books and left them on their doorstep for when they were ready to look at them. I couldn't make their pain go away, and I couldn't tell them how to grieve. But I could be there to listen and, as the mothers who had helped me had done, I could give them hope.

We went up to the fourth floor. Tammy was sitting at her desk and I could see the picture of a little boy over her shoulder. She saw me, stood up, and handed me the picture of her son. His name was Owen. I asked how she was holding up. She told me being at work and staying busy helped.

"I just *. . . I just miss him so much," she said and her eyes brimmed with tears. I put my arms around her and we just stood there like that, as the onlookers turned away.

She was three months into her grief. She had a long road ahead of her.

Lunch was a typical hospital conference meal: round tables covered with white tablecloths, a salad buffet, white meat or brown meat in sauce with gray mushrooms, green and orange vegetables, and a large basket of bread. Red was sitting at a table with a group of nurses surrounding him. What was it about this man, I wondered as I walked toward him. When he saw me, he stood up, smiled, and took the cowboy hat off the chair next to him.

He told me about his morning with the local politicians and, as I gobbled up my meat and vegetables, I noticed that the nurses were barely eating. Red Duke could not possibly have this affect on these nurses. Finally, I asked them why they weren't eating and as they picked at their lettuce leaves and eyed Red they told me that they were on Weight Watchers and tonight was weigh-in.

"What if you all started a walking club," I suggested. "You could walk on those pretty trails around the hospital after work or maybe before." They seemed to like that idea, though maybe they were just being polite and deep down were wondering who the heck I thought I was, suggesting that they walk around the hospital a bunch of times after they'd been on their feet all day. I had really no clue how mentally and physically taxing their jobs were, but I had a teeny tiny inkling. Everywhere I went I met nurses and I could tell that they were dedicated to their profession—the profession of healing. I admired them.

After lunch, Dr. Finley led Red and me to the conference room, where seats were filling up and people from other hospitals around the state were signing in. Dr. Finley told me he was pleased with the numbers. "We've got a good show of doctors," he said.

When everyone was seated, Dr. Finley introduced me and I made my way to the podium. I told Josie's story, reliving every detail for them. I told them how no one paid attention. How no one had listened to each other, and no one had listened to me. I told them what it felt like to have Josie die in my arms.

"What if someone had listened? What if the doctors and residents had communicated better and realized her weight had dropped 15 percent in twenty-four hours? What if she had been given a simple drink of water? What if a patient-safety program had been in place? I believe if any one of these things had occurred, Josie would be alive today."

The story flowed from Josie's death to the creation of the Josie King Foundation and all the programs that the foundation is part of. I wanted them to know that I was not just *talking* about medical errors, I was *doing* something about it.

"Josie's story is just one," I told them. "Every year there are thousands and thousands of others just like hers. I can't solve these problems, but you can, and you can do it now. This is not like cancer, AIDS, or diabetes. We don't have to wait for a scientific breakthrough. We can start by accepting the fact that there is a problem. We can start by communicating better: listening to patients, listening to parents, and listening to each other." I thanked them for all of their good work, and I begged them to keep going.

I sat down, drained but knowing that I had completed what I had come here for, and thinking that maybe something good would come of it.

I was looking forward to listening to Red and finally learning just who he was. More importantly, I knew that if there were any doctors in the audience who were still not convinced about the need to improve patient safety, Red would sway them. After all, he seemed to be a Texas legend.

Red walked up to the podium as a screen behind him slid down the back wall and the lights dimmed. A tape rolled, showing clips from a television series and news segments that featured him. The audience burst into laughter. These clips were the bloopers from the shows. They laughed at the scene of Red being caught on camera cussing. They continued to laugh at the footage of Red lassoing a cow and getting dragged through manure. They laughed at the scenes of Texas children dressing up as Dr. Red Duke for Halloween. His accompanying commentary added to the hilarity of it all.

I laughed along with the crowd and, as the footage unfolded, I started to understand the full stature of this unassuming cowboy. This sixty-something-year-old man who had been calling me honey and darlin' all over town had also accomplished a great deal in the medical world. His tireless work on educating the public about health issues and his crusades against traumatic injury had brought him into serious consideration for the position of surgeon general in 1989. On top of all that, he was a freelance vet, a Texas wrangler, and a major supporter of many wildlife and environmental conservation groups. He was the former host of the nationally syndicated *Texas Health Reports* and the series *Bodywatch*. Red had an unbridled way of communicating with his patients and fellow nurses and doctors. There was no question about it—this man was adored by many, many people.

The audience was loving every minute of Red's presentation and I couldn't blame them: it was sheer entertainment. But as he lingered at the podium, my patience began to fade. When would the presentation segue into patient safety? I waited, looking at my watch as the time ticked away. He had five minutes left. It remained a comedy act until the bitter end and my heart sank, but I stood up and joined the audience in a standing ovation. I was dumbfounded, trying to understand why I had ever agreed to come here in the first place.

There was some handshaking and picture taking afterward. Nurses thanked me and told me they would continue their work in patient safety. I watched as the group of doctors conversed with Dr. Finley in the back of the room. I was fuming. I wanted to walk up to them and scream that my daughter had died because of doctors with big egos just like them. They were only here to be entertained. As they walked toward me I bent over to pack my bag so that I would not have to talk to them.

"You did a great job," Dr. Finley said, introducing me to the group of doctors. They thanked me and told me they appreciated my coming to Texas. As they walked away I wondered what was going through their heads. I was certain it was not, "let's create patient-safety solutions to make our hospitals safer, so that ninety-eight thousand people don't die every year." I was sure they were talking about what a great show Red had put on and how funny it had been. I turned to Dr. Finley and asked him what Red Duke's talk had to do with preventing medical errors. "He didn't even mention the words *patient safety*," I said.

"Here's the deal," he explained. "Red is a legend around here. I knew if I advertised the fact that he was going to be speaking, more people would show up. He was going to draw a bigger crowd than just you alone."

"You mean the doctors came because of Red?" I asked.

"Yes, but that's not what's important here," he said. "What's important is that those doctors who I just introduced you to will be joining us at our next meeting. They're on board. It was your story, Josie's story, that convinced them."

I got it. I understood now. It was all part of Dr. Finley's plan. Red was the bowl of M&M's in front of the display. He drew in the crowd, but once the doctors were there, they had no choice but to listen to me. I was okay with that. All I cared about was that those doctors would be at that next patient-safety meeting. It was over and now it was time to just enjoy the rest of the day at St. Michael's before we headed to the airport.

I gathered my belongings and spotted the CEO's pretty wife making her way toward me with a small pouch in her hand. "I know this might sound strange to you," she said, "but when I was getting ready to come hear you speak this morning, I got this message from God and, well, I just had to make you these." She handed me the little gold pouch.

I untied the satin strings and emptied a pretty pair of dangly crystal earrings onto my palm. She told me the crystals were from a chandelier that had hung in an old house in town. "They're for you, to remind you of your mission, and to remind you of Texarkana," she said.

I thanked her and I took out my gold hoops and put in the Texarkana crystals.

Red and I decided to head to the cafeteria for a cup of coffee. He told me I had done a "mighty fine" job.

"You were the one who made them laugh," I said.

"Well, I might have made them laugh, but you were the one who inspired those stubborn ol' docs to get involved," he said. "You should feel mighty proud."

The cafeteria was one of the nicest I had been in. It offered fresh fruit, Häagen-Dazs ice cream, and gourmet coffee. We ordered our coffee and sat at a table in the hospital atrium, with its high ceilings reaching up to the second floor. In the center of the atrium sat a pretty grand piano that was being played by an older man wearing work pants and a bow tie. I asked Red if the man was an employee of St. Michael's. He told me that he had been a patient a few years ago. "He plays every day at two p.m. It's nice for the people sitting around here, but he really does it for the patients who have rooms up there in the radiology department, the people who are getting their cancer treatments."

Our conversation flowed easily from one topic to another, as if we were old friends. I liked listening to him tell me about his life in Afghanistan, where he had moved to develop a medical center. He told me he loved the country and its people. "I saw some crazy stuff over there—camel bites, sword wounds, rare parasitic diseases. You name it, I saw it." I asked him why he hadn't stayed longer. "I've been to a lot of places that sure were nice," he told me. "But sweetheart, I'm a Texan, and we all come back to Texas."

I went to get myself a yogurt and as I approached the cashier, I saw Chris, the CEO, talking to another person in line. He seemed to know everyone's name, even the food servers. He paid for his tea and then told the cashier that he'd pay for everyone else in line. He spotted me and asked if he could join us. As we walked back to the table, I noticed that, once again, Red was surrounded by a group of people.

"What is it about him?" I asked.

"He's just Red Duke. You'll never meet another person like him," Chris responded.

I thanked him for paying for my yogurt and asked if he knew the name of every St. Michael's employee. "Almost," he said. "We're sort of like family. We look after each other."

We all sat around and listened to Red's stories and for a while I felt like a part of the St. Michael's family, too. I didn't want it to end but it was time to head to the airport. My flight was a few hours before Red's, but he decided he would come along with us for the ride. I was glad we would have a little more time together.

We were back at the white Chevrolet with Jeffrey at the wheel. Red suggested to Jay that he go ahead and take the front seat. "I'll sit back here with Sorrel," Red said as he winked at me. Jay gave me another big brother jab as he opened the front door.

We sped down the highway, windows down, and for a moment I imagined I was not a mother grieving the loss of her child, I was just a girl in a pickup truck with her cowboy at the wheel and nothing to worry about. Red pointed to a strip of blue flowers that lay between the highways. "Sweetheart, those are Texas bluebells," he said. "Up in the plains, there are fields and fields of them."

We unloaded our bags at the airport and Jay and I headed to the ticket counter as Red waited with our luggage. *Unbelievable,* I thought, as I watched people walk past Red, do a double take, walk a few paces back, snap a photo on their cell phone, and then make a call.

"You'll never believe who's at the airport: Red Duke! Hell yeah, he's sitting right across from me."

Red seemed totally oblivious to it all.

A group of women sat down near him, trying to decide who was going to walk over to him first. I took my ticket from the agent and walked back over to him. He handed me a slip of paper with his phone number and address, which I put in my pocket.

"Will you be back east any time soon?" I asked.

"Nah, I gotta stick close to home. I'm getting too old for all of this," he said. "You come on back to Texas and I'll show you around. You can bring that Jay, too, he's a good ol' boy," he said, looking at Jay, who was fumbling with his belongings.

Our flight was beginning to board and Red and I stood up. He hugged me and whispered in my ear. "Now, listen to me," he said. "You keep up that work of yours, and don't you quit."

As I walked away, I glanced back at him. He waved until the airplane door closed and I realized with some sadness that I might never see him again. Maybe I was just one of the many women he had had this effect on. But in my own little world, I believed that he and I shared something more, a unique sort of bond. We were two misfits in the health care world, a world we both so desperately wanted to change. Maybe it was the idea of him that appealed to me most—

the strong, weathered cowboy-surgeon who had the guts to change the rules and fight for what he believed in. He taught me to be like a true cowboy and not back down.

As the plane sped down the runway, I decided that it wasn't just Red but all of Texarkana that had gotten to me. The wonderful nurses who worked themselves to the bone every day; Sister Damian, whose wise words I still recall often; Chris Karam, the young CEO, who really did care about his employees and patient safety; the doctors who let themselves be moved. I realized that big magical things are happening in little hospitals, in little towns, across America. As the plane lifted off and I watched the green fields of Texas fade away, I touched my crystal chandelier earrings, glad I had a piece of Texarkana to take home.

Powder Days

I try to imagine Josie if she were alive today. She would be seven, in second grade. Perhaps her short brown hair would be long now, pulled back in a pretty braid. Maybe she and Eva would share a room. I try to imagine her playing with her siblings, being a part of our family as it is now, but every time I close my eyes, my mind comes up blank. I wish I could picture her, but I can't. Maybe that's the way the mind works, making it hard to imagine what life *would* have been like; it keeps pushing us forward instead, moving us along, preventing us from spending too much time looking back.

I'd like to think that perhaps we would have had a fifth child anyway—that Sam was always going to be a part of our lives, but I don't know. One thing I do know is that I never would have fallen into the health care industry without Josie. I never would have become a part of the world of patient safety. Perhaps I would have been the mother I always thought I should be: the mother who cooked delicious meals, made homemade cupcakes on birthdays, and who attended every school field trip. And then, when the children were in school full time, perhaps I would have been the mother who did something fun and creative, like returning to the world of fashion design.

But none of that happened. Josie never got to play on a swing set. She never got to wear her hair in braids. She never got to kiss a boy. She never got to become a woman and have a family of her own.

And so I buy the cupcakes at the grocery store on the way to school. I pick up dinners at Let's Dish and serve them hot, making it look as if I whipped together a delicious, home-made meal. I stick to one field trip a year per child, always the quickest, easiest one: the trip to the tulip garden. I skip the coffees and teas organized by the other mothers. And when the children are at school I work.

People think that the Josie King Foundation is huge, with millions of dollars, occupying a large office space and em-ploying dozens of people. The truth is, we are a small grass-roots organization. The money comes from DVD donations, my speaking honorariums, corporate sponsors, Care Jour-nal sales, and donations from hundreds of people who care— because they want our health care system to be safer and because they believe the Josie King Foundation can help achieve that goal.

We have board members now: Rick Kidwell, who was the risk manager at Hopkins when Josie died and who later became my friend; Paul Bekman, our lawyer who has always taken an interest in the Josie King Foundation and helped the many families I have sent his way; Dr. Karen Frush, from Duke Medical Center, whose background as a nurse and ER doctor and whose passion for patient safety are making a huge difference in our health care system; and Dr. Peter Pronovost, who has become known worldwide for his con-tribution to patient safety and quality and was one of *Time* magazines one hundred most influential people in the world in 2008—soon thereafter he received a MacArthur "genius" grant. Each board member comes from a different background and brings a different perspective, and each is passionate about improving patient safety.

Rather than a large fancy office building, the Josie King Foundation occupies a single room in our house, a room whose walls are covered with my children's artwork. For years I ran the foundation by myself, but as it grew I could hardly keep up with all that needed to be done. I had barely enough time to work on new projects and initiatives, and felt that the quality of my work was slipping. I desperately needed help, and there was only one person I trusted enough to take over some of the responsibilities.

Andrea Wesol had been volunteering her time—nights and weekends—and handling DVD requests, helping correspond with organizations that wanted me to speak, and returning e-mails until finally I told her enough was enough. She had to let me pay her.

When Andrea was eight, her youngest brother Ryan was hospitalized for a brain tumor. Two and a half years later he died. She was passionate about the health care industry and helping it become safer. We worked well together. She was slow, methodical, and extremely organized. I was the complete opposite. She agreed to quit her job and work with me full time.

Because of Andrea, the Josie King Foundation is thriving and growing, with many exciting projects on the horizon, and because of Andrea I am sleeping a little bit better at night.

It has taken me a long time to balance my life as a patient-safety advocate and my life as a mother. After 3:30, when the children come home from school, I try not to answer the phone or look at the computer. If I don't want to travel to a hospital to give a speech, I say no. If it takes me three days to return an e-mail, it's okay. I might be a little slack on making delicious dinners, I could probably spend a little more time at the grocery store, and the house could be a little cleaner, but I do the best I can. My family is okay with it, and so am I.

I owe a lot to Gloria, too. As I got busier and busier with my patient-safety work she helped with the grocery shopping, the laundry, cleaning the house, and feeding the pets. She and I still have lunch together every day and she still tells me what to do. "Fix your hair, you can't go out like that . . . Take that shirt off and let me iron it . . . Don't wear those baggy pants, they make you look plump." Most of the time, I do as she says. Sometimes we argue, and it's usually over which one of us is going to pick up the dead bird, the dead chipmunk, or the half-eaten baby rabbit that the cat decided to bring into the house. But no matter what excuse I have, she always wins. She hands me a broom and dust pan and tells me, "go on girl and do your job," as she stands with her arms crossed, watching me. "Throw it in those trees over there," she says, pointing to the woods on the other side of the lawn.

When Sam comes home from school she chases him around the kitchen. "I missed my baby today," she says, capturing him and kissing him as he tries to wiggle out of her arms. I tell her she can't quit until Sam gets married.

I am six years into my grief and don't really consider myself a grieving mother anymore. Rather, I am simply continuing on the journey. Those first few years, I hardly ever let the children out of my sight thinking that someone was going to get in a car accident, someone was going to get cancer, or someone was going to be crushed by a falling tree. My fear of losing what I had left controlled me and it took years for me to realize that I had to let that fear go. But there are still times when I hear or see an ambulance driving toward the school, or when the phone rings late at night, or when the mother who was driving the kids home is an hour late, when those horrible feelings of panic flood back to me and my heart sinks, my mouth goes dry, my hands become clammy, my mind races, and I fear the very worst.

A surprisingly high percentage of married couples who lose a child end up divorced. We did not, but we had our moments. Tony and I grieved differently and it took me a long time to accept that. I had to let my pain out. I had to talk about it over and over again. I had to cry and wallow in it. I had to read books about losing a child. Tony did none of those things. I hardly ever saw him cry and he didn't want to read the grief books. He didn't want to talk about it. As I spent my nights tossing and turning, he slept soundly.

His different way of dealing with Josie's death confused me. One day, not long after Josie had died, I was sitting in the driver's seat of his car trying to figure out how to turn on the lights when I saw it: taped to the console was a picture of Tony kissing Josie. The pain of seeing her face shot through my heart and I ripped the photo off and stuck it in the glove compartment.

I backed out of the driveway, threw the car into drive, and turned the music on to get my mind off of what I had just seen. It wasn't his usual John Prine, the Mavericks, or the Grateful Dead coming through the speakers, though, it was "Baby Beluga."

Baby beluga in the deep blue sea
Swim so wild and you swim so free.

I listened to the words that I had not heard since I was last in the car with Josie. My eyes stung and I felt sick to my stomach. I ejected the CD and held it in my hand, wanting to throw it like a Frisbee to the back of the car, wanting it to smash against the window and break into a thousand pieces. How could he do this? How could this possibly make him feel better? I leaned over and shoved it in the glove compartment with the picture.

I didn't tell him what I had done until the next morning when he called me from his cell phone on his way to work. He asked where the picture and CD were. I told him they were in the glove compartment.

"Why'd you do that?"

"Because that stuff doesn't help," I said.

"Well, it helps me. When I go to work, and when I drive home, that's my only time to think about her. I don't have all day like you. I like looking at her picture and I like listening to that song. It reminds me of her. That's all I have."

As I listened to him, I realized that I had done something terribly selfish.

I wondered if he cried as he drove to work.

Sandra had always told me that men and women grieve differently and I was slowly beginning to realize that she was right. We each had to find our own way through this. If he didn't want to talk about it, I needed to respect that. We stuck by each other when sometimes it might have been easier to run away and, in the end, I believe our marriage has become stronger, simply because it survived the very worst.

My children kept me on board. In the beginning, they were the only reason I got out of bed. I had to make them lunches. I had to take them to school. I had to make them dinner and tie their shoes. I remember three-year-old Eva coming down one morning for breakfast as we prepared for school. She was wearing pink shorts with five fluorescent Band-Aids on each leg, perfectly aligned. For months I had not laughed, but that day, that moment, Eva with her fluorescent Band-Aids showed me that I could laugh again.

Jack is thirteen now, a full-fledged teenager. Not long ago, when Tony was out of town on business, Relly came running into my room at bedtime, telling me she had heard something on the third floor. I told her it was just the wind rattling the windows.

"Go back to sleep," I said.

Soon after, I heard all four children talking. I started down the hall but stopped to listen to their conversation.

"Relly and Eva, you guys stay here with Sam. I'm going up," I heard Jack say.

I peered around the corner, not letting them see me, and watched Jack, holding the wooden baseball bat that he had made at camp, creep slowly up the steps to the dark and cavernous third floor. Relly, Eva, and Sam sat scrunched up together against the wall with their slippers sticking out from beneath their bathrobes, holding their breaths.

Jack came trotting down the stairs. "It was just a window that blew open. It's closed now," he told them. "Let's get back in bed."

"Phew," Relly said. "Come on, Eva, let's go."

"Sam, you can sleep with me if you want," Jack said.

I tiptoed back to my room, not wanting to interrupt the happy scene that had just occurred.

I know that Jack will take care of his siblings if ever we're not around. When he graduated from the lower school he was awarded the "Unsung Hero" award, a recognition for the student who quietly helps others. I don't know if he's like that because of Josie, or if it is just from being the oldest child. I'd like to think that Josie gives all our children extra strength to go beyond the call of duty, to do things that may sometimes seem difficult.

Relly is almost twelve and in sixth grade, and Josie's death is not a part of her everyday existence. It is not a part of any of the children's everyday existence. Every once in a while, though, I stumble across a picture of Josie that Relly put into a special frame that she made or taped into a journal. Sometimes we talk about Josie. I ask her if she remembers her and she says, "Yeah, a little bit."

Each of them, I believe, is a bit of an old soul. They are a little wiser. They are a little more sensitive. They survived and they helped their parents survive. I may never know the full extent to which Josie's death has affected their lives but I figure when the time is right, they will tell me. They were so young when she died: six, five, and three. Sometimes I am glad that they were that young and can't really remember, but most of the time I wish they had had just a little more time with her.

Sam is five and understands that he once had a big sister named Josie, who died before he was born. We are all grateful to have him in our lives. He brought us together and kept us moving forward as a family. In time, he will understand the details and will know what our family once was, but for now, he knows as much as a five-year-old needs to know.

I owe so much to each of them: Jack, Relly, Eva, and Sam. They gave me a reason to live when I was in my darkest moments and one day I will tell them how they saved my life.

They say that time heals. I don't believe that anyone can ever *fully* heal after losing a child, but time does help. It's really the only thing that lessens the pain: the weeks, the months, the years. I don't cry anymore when I talk about her. I don't think about her every minute of the day. The children can bring up her name and not have to worry about their mother bursting into tears.

We don't have long serious conversations about Josie, and we still don't have any pictures of her around the house. I am sure my old therapist Sandra, whom I have not seen in a number of years, would tell me it's wrong. But when I look into Josie's eyes, my chest still hurts and my eyes still sting. I don't worry too much about the lack of photos, because she is all over my desk, my computer, and my BlackBerry. Her photos may not be splashed around our house, but she is everywhere, and her siblings know it. They see it in the work I do and that, I believe, is what keeps her alive.

Someone once told me that the death of a child is like having a huge tree ripped out of the ground: it leaves a big, empty, gaping hole. But gradually, over time, ferns, flowers, and little trees start growing, filling the hole. Josie's death left a painful hole in my heart that will always be there, but things are filling it—the Josie King Foundation, the wonderful people I have met in the health care industry, and the knowledge that Josie's story is making our health care system safer and, most beautiful of all, that her death is saving lives.

I've learned that life doesn't always work out the way you had planned. You learn to adapt to what is thrown your way, and you make the most of it. Our kids did not grow up skiing the great mountains of Lake Tahoe as I dreamed. We have settled for the ski hills of Pennsylvania, a little place called Roundtop, where you can smell bacon and eggs frying in the morning as you load the Minuteman chairlift.

Tony and I wait at the bottom of the slalom course, leaning against our poles as Sam makes snowballs. We look up and squint into the sun trying to catch a glimpse of Relly at the top section of the course, tearing down the hill in search of the steepest and fastest line to get her around the gates and through the finish. Her brother Jack, above, watches her closely, strategizing to make sure his sister does not beat him. Her blonde ponytail whizzes past us as she tucks her body and throws her arms forward over the finish line and the cow bells ring. We can see Eva's red helmet move toward the starting gate. Waiting for Jack and Eva, watching the other racers come down the hill, I hear Van Morrison's "Bright Side of the Road" coming through the outdoor speakers.

I breathe in the cold air and feel the warm sun on my face. It's perfect, all of it: the snow, our little mountain in Pennsylvania, my family. This is it. This is how it was all meant to be. I look up at the sky and I know Josie is smiling down on us making this a perfect day.

I never thought I could say the words that my friend Rachel, whose son died three years before Josie, said to me so many years ago. But I can, now. We are happy. We are profoundly happy. We have seen the dark side; we have been there. We have lived it and we have survived. It has taken a long time to find that happiness again, but I've got it, and I'm holding on tight.

Acknowledgments

For many months Josie and her story swirled around in my head, sometimes keeping me up at night until I would turn on the light and let it out on paper. At times it seemed to write itself.

One day I took my bits and pieces of writing to the Ivy Bookshop and showed it to a saleslady. Her name was Shirley Fergenson and she was the first person who told me I had a different kind of voice and that I could write. She pushed me, she encouraged me, she told me to not give up. Without her this book never would have been written and I thank her.

Thank you Jane Roessner for reading Josie's story early on and for putting me in contact with the publishing world. Thank you Deanne Urmy for giving me a 101 on how the world of publishing works. "Find an agent," you said, and you showed me how. Thank you Christy Fletcher, my agent. "Write a proposal," you said, and you showed me the way. Thank you Lynette Clemetson.

Thank you Grove/Atlantic: Joan Bingham, my editor, her assistant Alex Littlefield, Deb Seager, Morgan Entrekin, and to everyone else at Grove. From the beginning you saw this as a book that was about more than a child dying, a book that could help others. Thank you for making a difference in ways that I never could have on my own.

I'd like to thank all of my wonderful health care industry friends who have done so much for patient safety and who have supported me in sharing Josie's story: Dr. Don Berwick, Madge Kaplan, and Jonathan Small of IHI. Thank you to my friends at Johns Hopkins: Dr. Peter Pronovost, Dr. George Dover, Dr. David Cromwell, Dr. Marlene Miller, Dr. Lauren Bogue, Dr. Albert Wu, Laurie Rome, Kim Hoppe, and Joann Rodgers. Thank you to Dr. Charles Paidas, Dr. Milissa McKee, and Dr. Amal Murarka's wife, Dr. Marjorie Rosenthal, for letting me share our story. Thank you, Dr. Chuck Denham who still sends me hundreds of DVDs so that Josie's story can continue to make a difference. Thanks to Dr. Karen Frush, Tami Merryman, Chris Goeschel, Linda Kenney, Dr. Rick van Pelt, Dr. Red Duke, and Richard Boothman. Thanks, too, to Erika Niedowski and Sandra Fink. Of course, thanks to Dale Ann Micalizzi and Julie Koleszar. Justin and Charlotte will not be forgotten.

A special thank you to Rick Kidwell and Paul Bekman. The day Tony and I signed the settlement papers, I told you both that you'd never get rid of me. Thank you for your help with the Josie King Foundation and for supporting this book but most of all thank you for helping me help others.

Andrea Wesol has been with me every step of the way. Her calmness, her brilliance, her organized way kept it all together for me, and for the Josie King Foundation. She understood my vision for this book, and she pushed me until she got it out of me. We argued until she won and usually she was right. Without Andrea I may have given up on the book. Without Andrea I may have given up on the foundation. I thank her for never giving up on me and most of all I thank her for her quiet humble contribution to the world of patient safety.

Thank you to my friends who helped me throughout. Thank you Gloria for traveling down the road with me and for picking up the pieces. To my siblings Mac, Mary Earle, and Margaret, and to my wonderful parents. A special thanks to Jay King, my brother-in-law, for letting me convince him that he needed to join me in this world of patient safety. Thank you for all of your hard work and for doing so much to help improve patient safety and for reading this book more times than you would have liked to.

Some people tell me I have made a difference, that I have made health care safer, but the truth of the matter is that there are so many other people, so many great organizations that are doing amazing things to make our health care system safer. Besides the people and the organizations I have mentioned in this book I'd like to thank Dr. Lucian Leape, Sue Sheridan, Dr. Atul Gawande, Dr. Robert Wachter, the World Health Organization, the National Patient Safety Foundation, and the Robert Wood Johnson Foundation. Thank you to all of the medical and nursing school students who have heard me tell Josie's story. Thank you to all of the wonderful statewide organizations, hospital and healthcare systems that invited me in, listened to Josie's story and did something to become safer. Thank you to all the CEOs who insist on making patient safety a priority. And most of all thank you to the wonderful doctors, nurses, and other health care providers who work hard each day to prevent the next error from happening. You are the ones who are making a difference. You are the ones who make health care safer for us all and for that I am eternally grateful.

I would like to thank the nurses at Hopkins who cared for Josie—especially the nurses on the sixth floor. Since writing this book I have learned more about your efforts to help Josie the night before she arrested. Thank you for trying so hard.

Lastly and most importantly I thank my children Jack, Relly, Eva, and Sam, who have seen a phone that sometimes seems to be attached to my head, or my face that seems to always be in front of a computer screen more often than I care to admit. Thank you for letting me do what I needed to do. And most of all I thank Tony. Always, always, always calm, always with good advice, and each time I said I want to give up you pushed me back out there.

I am lucky and thankful to have the memory of a pretty little girl named Josie whose spirit is with me every day and who will always be my inspiration.

Resource Guide

Since Josie's death we have tried to do our small part in helping patients, their families, and health care providers.

This resource guide is divided into two parts. The first part is for patients and their families and consists of tips on how to manage a stay at the hospital, along with advice on what to do when an unexpected event occurs.

The second part of the resource guide is for health care professionals and consists of tips from my perspective, that of a patient or family member, on how to continue to provide safe and effective care. While this guide has made a distinction between patients and health care professionals, the resources listed in either section will be of interest to everybody who wants to learn more about patient safety.

I have asked a few expert friends of mine to share their advice, but remember, this is general information, not formal legal advice. It is best to discuss the particulars of your individual situation with your trusted health care team.

—Sorrel King, January 2009
The Josie King Foundation
www.josieking.org

Part One: For the Patient and Family

The first and most important thing to remember when you are at the hospital is that you are in good hands. Trust the doctors and nurses who are taking care of you. Have faith that they will do the very best they can in caring for you. At the same time, you should also stay on top of the medical information that you will receive. Here are a few things that we, as patients or patient advocates, can do to stay safe and organized while we are at the hospital:

1. Take a NOTEBOOK with you to keep track of information. The Josie King Foundation can provide you with a Care Journal. For more information, please visit www.josieking.org.
2. Give your health care team the FULL INFORMATION ABOUT YOUR HEALTH and tell them what medications you take, your personal habits—like alcohol use or smoking—your diet, and any allergies you may have.
3. It is always nice to know the NAMES of the doctors and nurses who are taking care of you. Use your notebook to keep track.
4. Make sure everyone who comes into the room WASHES THEIR HANDS. Not only do caregivers need to wash their hands but so do family members and anyone who comes into the room and may have contact with the patient.
5. Don't be afraid to SPEAK UP. If something doesn't seem right to you, trust your instincts.
6. Always, always ASK QUESTIONS if there is something you do not understand.

7. Be grateful. SAY THANK YOU to the doctors and nurses who take care of you.
8. Try to RELAX.

What to do when there is an unexpected outcome.

I have asked two legal experts to provide some advice. If you have read this book you already know of Rick Kidwell and Paul Bekman. Rick is the head of risk management at UPMC, the University of Pittsburgh Medical Center. Paul is a medical malpractice lawyer at Salsbury, Clements, Bekman, Marder and Adkins, LLC in Baltimore, Maryland. Here are their answers to some common questions:

Q. To whom within the hospital should a patient or loved one talk when they believe a mistake may have been made?

Rick: You should start with the doctors and nurses taking care of you or your family member. Tell them your concerns in a nonconfrontational, nonaccusatory way. Ask them to explain what has happened, and why, and what will be done to help you or the patient get better.

Paul: Rick's response is a good one. It is always best to deal firsthand with the people who have direct responsibility for the patient. In the event that you do not get satisfaction, you should contact the risk management office, or even the legal department to express your concerns.

Q. What should be done if their concerns are being ignored?

Rick: Ask to speak to the nurse manager and the division/department chief. If that doesn't work, ask to talk to patient relations so you can file a grievance, which hospital regulations require be responded to. You could also ask to meet with the risk manager or hospital counsel if the patient relations route does not work.

Q. If a patient or family member wants medical records, how do they go about retrieving them?

Rick: The patient or family member should send a written request to the hospital's records department, requesting the records. Local laws usually give hospitals a few weeks to copy and send the records. Keep in mind that there will be a delay if you ask for records while the patient is still in the hospital because the chart probably won't be copied until after the patient has been discharged. The hospital does not want to interrupt access to the records by taking a chart away to be copied while the patient is still in the hospital. You may also ask your attending physician to go over the chart with you while you or your family member is in the hospital if you need immediate access to the chart. The hospital will require a caregiver be with you while you review the chart, to answer questions and to keep the chart in order.

Paul: I agree with Rick as to medical records. Many times a hospital may be reluctant to release a patient's medical records, particularly if the patient is still in the hospital. It is therefore likely that you will not be able to get a complete set of medical records until such time as the patient has been discharged from the hospital, but it is absolutely *essential* to get all the medical records pertaining to the patient's care. What all of the records consist of may not be known to the person requesting them. If you believe that you have a legitimate claim, and the issue is getting a complete set of records, it may be advisable to consult with counsel even if it is for the limited purpose of obtaining a complete set of medical records.

Q. At what point should patients and their families consider hiring a lawyer?

Paul: The decision to hire a lawyer is a personal one. Different people may be motivated by different considerations when they think about hiring a lawyer. The first concern should be the care and treatment of the patient in making sure that the patient receives optimal care under the best possible circumstances. If, in fact, it is believed that a mistake has been made, it would be advisable to consult with an attorney to have them explain what the patient's legal rights are. Many times a phone call can be made by counsel to the hospital to clear up any problems that have developed. On the other hand, it may be necessary to obtain medical records in order to evaluate whether, in fact, there is a viable claim that should be pursued. In any event, it is absolutely essential that if medical records are obtained that *all* of the medical records must be requested and obtained.

Rick: I agree with Paul. Circumstances will help steer the patient or family to the appropriate time to retain counsel.

Q. What is the best way to find a reputable lawyer?

Paul: There are many different ways to obtain counsel. In any particular city, there is usually a recognized group of individuals who do medical negligence work. It would be very easy to go to a reference such as Martindale Hubbell, which is a law directory, but that will give you only basic information. Some of the more comprehensive sources that you could consult are the following:

- Best Lawyers in America (www.bestlawyers.com)
- American Board of Trial Advocates (www.abota.org)
- American College of Trial Lawyers (www.actl.com)
- International Academy of Trial Lawyers (www.iatl.net)
- International Society of Barristers (www.international societyofbarristers.org)
- The various local magazines around the country that have identified the so-called Super Lawyers, or top 5 percent of attorneys, in that particular jurisdiction.

It is essential in medical negligence suits to obtain not just any lawyer but a lawyer who concentrates his or her practice in the medical negligence area.

Q. How many lawyers should the patient or family interview?

Paul: This is a matter of personal choice. Sometimes it may be one interview. Other times, just like any other serious decision that a person would make, it is a good idea to interview several individuals. It is important for those who are seeking counsel to be comfortable with the lawyer that they choose. This relates not only to competence, but in terms of being able to work with that particular person in what is likely to be an extremely emotional and difficult time.

Q. How does the patient or family know if they have found the right lawyer?

Paul: This is largely a matter of comfort. You will generally know, particularly if you have engaged in the interview process, who the right lawyer is for you. There are many fine and competent lawyers who practice in the area of medical negligence, many of whom would be more than capable and able to handle a particular case.

Q. When something goes wrong and the family feels they are being ignored by the hospital, they may want to get the media involved. What are your thoughts on that?

Paul: My personal view is that there will be plenty of time later to involve the media if it is necessary.

What needs to be done initially is to find out the facts and determine whether or not you have a viable case. This has to be done with good, hard work and preparation. Once a case is filed it becomes a public record and can then be subject to media interest. It is my practice not to involve the media and, instead, try to do the best job that I can for my clients.

Rick: I think the urge to run to the media should be suppressed while you try to work things out directly with the hospital and nurses and doctors. First, you need to make sure you have all the facts. Second, you should give the hospital and its staff a chance to do the right thing. Third, if there is to be a claim or litigation, you've lost some leverage if you've already played the publicity card.

Q. If a family who has been affected by medical errors wants to partner with the hospital to try to accomplish some good, how would you recommend they go about this? Where should they start? Who should they talk to?

Rick: Again, the best place to start is with the doctors and nurses. Let them know you want to help them improve care. You could also ask to speak to the risk manager with the same offer.

Other Resources

There are many resources on patient safety. These are a few Web sites and books that we recommend.

Web sites

Agency for Healthcare Research and Quality (AHRQ)
www.ahrq.gov
Sponsored by the U.S. Department for Health and Human Services, this is the United States' lead federal agency for research on health care quality, costs, outcomes, and patient safety. Among many other things, this Web site offers information regarding funding opportunities, nursing research, and health-service research findings for policy makers.

Pages of particular interest to patients and their families include:

> 20 Tips to Help Prevent Medical Errors
> http://www.ahrq.gov/consumer/20tips.htm

> 20 Tips to Help Prevent Medical Errors in Children
> http://www.ahrq.gov/consumer/20tipkid.htm

> Other safety resources for patients and their families
> http://www.ahrq.gov/consumer/index.html#quality

Institute for Family-Centered Care
www.familycenteredcare.org
This nonprofit organization promotes collaborative relationships among patients, families, and health care professionals. The institute accomplishes its mission through training, teaching tools, and information dissemination as well as through research and public policy initiatives.

The Joint Commission
www.jointcommission.org

The Joint Commission provides evaluation and accreditation services for many organizations including general, psychiatric, children's and rehabilitation hospitals, nursing homes, and other long-term-care facilities. Through accreditation it is hoped that facilities will continuously improve the safety and quality of care provided to the public. Patients can report health care-related grievances through the Joint Commission at http://www.jointcommission.org/GeneralPublic/Complaint.

The Josie King Foundation
www.josieking.org

We keep our Web site up to date with the latest information on patient safety. You will learn tips on how to stay safe in medical settings, patient safety news, and activities of the Josie King Foundation. We also host a message board where patients and families can post their stories, ask their questions, answer other people's questions, and otherwise discuss patient-safety issues. I also have a blog that I post to every now and then.

Medically Induced Trauma Support Services (MITSS)
www.mitss.org

MITSS is a nonprofit organization that works to support patients, families, and medical professionals who have been affected by a medical error. Its projects include support groups, advocacy opportunities, and a telephone hotline.

Persons United Limiting Substandards and Errors in Health Care (PULSE)
www.pulseamerica.org

PULSE is a nonprofit organization dedicated to reducing medical errors through providing a supportive network to connect people who have been affected by medical errors, educating the public to raise awareness, and advocating for an improved health care system.

Books

To Err Is Human: Building a Safer Health System, by the Institute of Medicine. Washington, DC: National Academies Press, 2000.

This seminal report by the Institute of Medicine seriously examines problems in the health care arena and proposes a national plan to reduce medical errors.

Complications: A Surgeon's Notes on an Imperfect Science, by Atul Gawunde. New York: Henry Holt and Company, 2002.

Surgical resident and author Gawunde explores the fallibility of doctors and the imprecision of medicine and technology as well as the humanity of the medical profession.

Wall of Silence, by Rosemary Gibson and Janardan Prasad Singh. Washington, DC: Lifeline Press, 2003.

Gibson and Singh recant numerous stories of victims of medical malpractice and highlight the grave mistakes that occur daily in our health care system.

How Doctors Think, by Jerome Groopman. New York: Houghton Mifflin, 2007.

Groopman explores both how and why most doctors get health care practices right, and how and why they sometimes get it wrong.

The Best Practice: How the New Quality Movement Is Transforming Medicine, by Charles Kenney. New York: PublicAffairs, 2008.

Kenney details the history of the modern patient-safety movement and shows how safety leaders have brought about great improvements in health care delivery.

You: The Smart Patient: An Insider's Handbook for Getting the Best Treatment, by Michael F. Roizen and Mehmet C. Oz. New York: Free Press, 2006.

This is an indispensable handbook that can help everyone get the best health care possible. A must-have for anyone about to enter the hospital.

Questions Patients Need to Ask, by David J. Shulkin. Philadelphia: Xlibris, 2008.

The CEO of Beth Israel Medical Center in New York City collects questions that patients should ask their health care team in order to get safe care and be as informed as possible when in the hospital or in any health care setting.

Internal Bleeding: The Truth Behind America's Terryifying Epidemic of Medical Mistakes, by Robert Wachter and Kevin Shojania. New York: Rugged Land, 2005.

University of California San Francisco School of Medicine professors analyze case studies to emphasize how faulty systems—rather than individuals—are to blame for the epidemic of medical errors.

Understanding Patient Safety, by Robert Wachter. New York: McGraw-Hill Professional, 2007.

An excellent primer on the field of patient safety—

principles, types of errors, case studies, key statistics, and solutions.

Part Two: For the Health Care Provider

This section of the resource guide is for anybody who works in a health care setting. Modern health care delivery consists of many elements: cutting-edge scientific knowledge, mastery of procedures, and diagnostic arts, to name but a few. Communication—with patients and their families, but also among colleagues—is essential to a safe health care system. Here are a few tips from my perspective:

1. LISTEN to the patient and family.
2. LISTEN to each other.
3. Use *The Josie King Story* DVD to inspire your coworkers to create a culture of safety. For more information, please visit www.josieking.org.
4. Consider programs like CONDITION HELP: patient- and family-activated rapid response teams. For more information on Condition Help, visit www.josieking .org or contact UPMC. We'll help you get started.
5. Encourage your patients and/or their family members to keep track of information by WRITING information down. Some hospitals have partnered with the Josie King Foundation to give the Care Journal to their admitted patients as a gift. To learn more about this program, please visit www.josieking.org.
6. Develop and practice essential health care COMMUNICATION SKILLS, from how to communicate with coworkers to how to disclose a medical error to a patient or his or her family.

7. If you are involved in medical education, consider advocating for the increased discussion of medical errors and communication skills in the MEDICAL TRAINING CURRICULUM.

8. Familiarize yourself with the DISCLOSURE POLICIES at the hospitals and medical care facilities at which you work.

9. Encourage your patients and their family members to PARTNER with you in their care.

What to do when there has been an unexpected outcome.

A medical error that causes harm to a patient is a devastating event for the patient, their loved ones, and the doctors, nurses, and other medical professionals that helped care for the patient. Here again, Rick Kidwell and Paul Bekman share their opinions on how to deal with these issues.

Q. When a doctor or nurse makes a mistake, what is your advice to them? Should they apologize right off or do they need to talk to the risk manager at their organization before they do anything?

Rick: The doctor or nurse should notify risk management, if possible, before apologizing because he or she—I hope—hasn't had experience dealing with this situation but the risk manager probably has. The risk manager can offer advice about how best to disclose, including who should do so, and can help determine what will be done to analyze the error to try to prevent a recurrence. The risk manager may also be able to offer financial considerations for the patient or family to help get them through the effects of an error. That said, however, it is more important that the doctors and nurses communicate with the patients and their families and not delay any needed discussion to track down risk management. Risk management will support the doctor or nurse who does the right thing by apologizing, explaining, and assuring the patient and family.

Paul: I think it is extremely important that a line of communication be developed between the patient and the hospital staff, whether this be with the doctors who are caring for the patient, the risk management office, or the legal department. Open lines of communication should exist to enhance the partnership relationship. In many states an apology for a medical error is not admissible in subsequent proceedings. Some states have recently passed laws that permit a doctor or hospital to apologize for a medical mistake. It is my view that a doctor will reduce his chances of having a medical negligence case filed against him or her if he or she is open and honest about a mistake being made.

Q. What advice would you give a hospital that does not have a full disclosure policy?

Rick: Every hospital should have that policy. Regulations require it but, more importantly, it is the right thing to do. I would advise any hospital that doesn't have such a policy to look at this as just another phase of what should be ongoing communication between patients/families and doctors/nurses.

Q. Has there been any research done on the relationship between disclosure or apology on the part of the health care provider and malpractice lawsuits?

Rick: There are some studies, including a recent one from Harvard that concludes that disclosure may actually increase the number of claims and/or dollars spent in lawsuits. Other studies reach a different result—that disclosure may actually prevent lawsuits. It really doesn't matter which view is accurate; what does matter is that disclosure is the right thing to do, regardless of legal ramifications.

Paul: My advice would be to make a disclosure as soon as possible after an error occurs. This will enhance the patient's trust of the physician and in many cases may be the main factor in having the patient not proceed with a medical negligence claim. As far as research is concerned relating to the relationship between disclosure and an apology after medical errors and malpractice suits, my experience has been anecdotal. Many times I will meet a patient who says that the doctor told them he or she made a mistake, but the patient thinks he or she has been a wonderful physician and does not want to bring an action against the doctor. On the other hand, there are many instances where an error may have resulted in a catastrophic event, such as serious personal injury or death. In those circumstances, although the apology has been made and the error admitted, these acts may enhance the resolution of the claim without having to undergo unnecessary and prolonged litigation.

Other Resources

Web sites

Agency for Healthcare Research and Quality (AHRQ)
www.ahrq.gov/qual/

Sponsored by the U.S. Department of Health and Human Services, this is the nation's lead federal agency for research on health care quality, costs, outcomes, and patient safety. Among many other subjects, this Web site offers information regarding funding opportunities, nursing research, and health-service research findings for policy makers.

American Society for Healthcare Risk Management (ASHRM)
www.ashrm.org

ASHRM is a membership group for risk managers in the American Hospital Association (AHA) with members representing health care, insurance, law, and other related professions. ASHRM promotes effective and innovative risk management strategies and professional leadership through education, advocacy, publications, networking, and interactions with leading health care organizations and government agencies. ASHRM initiatives focus on developing and implementing safe and effective patient-care practices, the preservation of financial resources, and the maintenance of safe working environments.

Institute for Healthcare Improvement (IHI)
www.ihi.org

This is a not-for-profit organization promoting the improvement of health care throughout the world. The Web site is designed for health care providers and organizations. The site contains work-space improvement tools, conferences and teaching programs, and a multitude of books, videos, and audio materials that can be used as teaching aids to promote patient safety and health care.

Robert Wood Johnson Foundation
www.rwjf.org

Ensuring that all Americans receive high-quality care is central to the mission of the Robert Wood Johnson Foundation (RWJF). It has placed a strong focus on improving the health and health care for all Americans, especially those with chronic conditions. The foundation's goals are to set national standards for quality, to track progress, and to reward successes. They offer funding opportunities to achieve this end.

The Joint Commission
www.jointcommission.org

The Joint Commission provides evaluation and accreditation services for many organizations including general, psychiatric, children's and rehabilitation hospitals, nursing homes, and other long-term-care facilities. Through accreditation it is hoped that facilities will continuously improve the safety and quality of care provided to the public.

The Josie King Foundation
www.josieking.org

Our Web site is regularly updated with the latest information available on patient safety. You can learn about patient-safety issues that affect your work and how to implement patient-safety programs at your hospital.

There are two pages on the Web site that would be of particular interest to doctors and nurses trying to cope with a medical error:

> CARE FOR THE CAREGIVER is a research project that we sponsored to investigate whether or not there are therapeutic benefits to guided writing exercises based on a medical error event specifically or the stress of the health care profession in general. The latest information on this project is available on the Web site under "Foundation Programs." An excerpt from the Nursing Journal is included in the Appendix of this book.

> CONNECTING WITH OTHERS is a bulletin board on which people interested in patient safety can communicate with each other, post questions and comments, answer questions, or discuss anything related to patient safety. We have a special section for medical professionals so they can specifically network with each other. You can find this section under "Resource Center."

The Leapfrog Group
www.leapfroggroup.org

The Leapfrog Group is a voluntary program aimed at promoting the fact that big leaps in health care safety, quality, and customer value will be recognized and rewarded. Among other initiatives, Leapfrog works with its members to encourage access to health care information and rewards for hospitals that have a proven record of high-quality care. For patients and families, there is consumer section on the Web site that allows one to see the safety ranking of the hospitals in your area. For hospitals, the site has a public reporting initiative and a rewards program.

Medically Induced Trauma Support Services (MITSS)
www.mitss.org
MITSS is a nonprofit organization that works to support patients, families, and medical professionals who have been affected by a medical error. Its projects include support groups, advocacy opportunities, and a telephone hotline.

National Patient Safety Foundation (NPSF)
www.npsf.org
The foundation's main goal is to improve the safety of patients through both education and raising public awareness. The Web site contains a wealth of information relating to research programs, safety awareness conferences, and patient-safety resource links. Additionally, there are discussion forums and a library with many resources.

The Patient Safety Group
www.patientsafetygroup.org
Sorrel King cofounded the Patient Safety Group with her brother-in-law Jay King to assist hospitals with their quality and safety improvement efforts. The Patient Safety Group's mission is to encourage a culture of safety by providing tools that allow health care organizations the ability to communicate, collaborate, improve, and share. The Patient Safety Group's initial program, eCUSP (electronic Comprehensive Unit-based Patient Safety Program), provides motivated care-

givers the opportunity to manage, monitor, organize, account for, and share their patient-safety efforts. The Patient Safety Group also provides a tool for measuring a hospital's culture of safety, a requirement that was mandated by the Joint Commission in 2008.

Removing Insult from Injury (Albert Wu's video on full disclosure)
www.jhsph.edu/removinginsultfrominjury

Dr. Albert Wu has created a training tool to help educate medical workers on how to disclose medical errors to patients and their families. You can learn more about the tool kit and order a copy on Dr. Wu's Web site.

Sorry Works!
www.sorryworks.net

This coalition serves to organize information, news, ideas, and research about the concept of "sorry works" and related full-disclosure efforts. There is information about states with "Sorry" laws as well as information about hospital and physician disclosure.

Books

Crossing the Quality Chasm: A New Health System for the 21st Century, by the Institute of Medicine. Washington, DC: National Academy Press, 2001.

In this follow-up to the seminal *To Err Is Human* report, the Institute of Medicine authors suggest solutions that can be implemented by the health care community to improve the American health care system.

Rapid Response Teams, second edition, by Della M. Lin. Marblehead, MA: HCPro, 2008.

This multimedia resource walks clinicians through the steps necessary to implement a successful rapid response team.

Error Reduction in Health Care, by Patrice L. Spath. San Francisco: Jossey-Bass, 2000.

Spath examines the causes of medical errors and offers health care providers suggestions about how to reduce mistakes.

Appendix—Excerpts from the Nursing Journal

A Writing Workbook to Help
Nurses Cope with Stress

The Josie King Foundation would like to thank all of the nurses who go to work each day with the intent of helping others. We recognize that along with experiencing the joys of healing, you are also faced with issues such as death and dying, pain and suffering, challenges with staff, complicated work environments related to new technologies, medical errors and near misses—all of which can lead to stress and burnout.

One way to cope with the stresses that come with being a nurse is to keep a journal: a place for you to unload your thoughts and feelings about work-related events that may be too difficult to talk about even with family and friends. With the help of nurses across the country, as well as with the collaboration of Dr. Janel Sexton, assistant professor at the Johns Hopkins Quality and Safety Research Group, the Josie King Foundation has created a specialized workbook journal for nurses. We are including excerpts here in the hope that they will inspire you to begin keeping a journal of your own, and to help you deal with the challenges you face every day.

We appreciate all that you do in the name of healing.

For more information on the *Nursing Journal,* please visit www.josieking.org.

—Sorrel King and the Josie King Foundation

Stress evaluation

Stress manifests itself in a wide variety of ways. We recommend that you review the list of stress-related symptoms before you begin the exercises. Record how often and how intensely you experience any of these symptoms. It's a good idea to cultivate an awareness of the signs of stress that you exhibit. It will also provide you with a simple baseline to reflect the various ways that stress affects you.

Physical Signs of Stress
Back pain
Chest pain
Exhaustion
Frequent colds
Headaches
Muscle pain
Neck/shoulder pain
Racing heart
Upset stomach

Intellectual Signs of Stress
Difficulty concentrating
Excessive worrying
Indecisiveness

Loss of interest in something that used to give you
 pleasure
Loss of sense of humor
Memory problems
Negative thinking

Behavioral Signs of Stress
Avoiding others
Blaming others
Changes in appetite (overeating or undereating)
Chronic absenteeism
Coming late to work
Inability to complete a task
Increased drug or alcohol use
Insomia
Lethargy
Nail biting
Procrastinating
Sleeping too much

Emotional Signs of Stress
Anger
Anxiety/fear
Feeling out of control
Feeling overwhelmed
Guilt
Irritability
Loneliness
Mood swings
Sadness

Guided journal entries

We have prepared some guided writing prompts to inspire your process. Each asks a question related to nursing; think about the question and write your response in your journal.

- Why did you become a nurse?
- What do you like best about being a nurse? What do you like least?
- Write about a specific patient who affected you.
- How does collaboration with others affect your work as a nurse?
- Write about a nursing accomplishment that makes you proud.

Writing guidelines

- Try to write in a quiet space without interruptions.
- Really let go and explore your very deepest emotions and thoughts.
- Don't worry about grammar, spelling, or sentence structure. Just write.

Self-guided writing

It is important to write about whatever is affecting you most. Has a medical error or near-miss affected the way you do your job? Are relationships with coworkers affecting your quality of work life? Are you confronting issues related to human pain and dying? Reflect on your work as a nurse, and write about the most pressing issues. Remember to go deep and really explore your deepest thoughts and emotions.

Tips from nurses on how to cope with stress

Great advice often comes from people who have experienced and coped with similar situations. We have gathered words of wisdom from nurses around the country on what they find helpful in dealing with the pressures of the profession.

"I find that in order to care well for others, I must first take care of myself. Without my health, I wouldn't have the strength to perform the hard work nursing requires. Daily exercise and good nutrition are essential to helping me cope with the stress. I love group fitness classes, weightlifting, and 'clean' eating!"—Kathryn A., BSN, RN, South Lyon, MI

"As a nurse practitioner I try to remember to always thank everyone for helping me to help my patients. It really is a group effort. And thanking people is a great way to defuse stress, as it makes people feel appreciated."—Kimberly B., MSN, CRNP, Pittsburgh, PA

"Take a moment every day to reflect on what went well, what didn't go so well, and what you can do better tomorrow. Always take a moment to take a deep breath when the world is moving quickly by and you can't keep up. Who knows? Your speed might be what everyone should be moving at throughout the day. Baking fresh treats for your coworkers is the best medicine and always makes a nurse's day brighter."
—Sheryl C., RN, MSN, Washington, DC

"Personally, I make sure I stay in contact with those I love the most during the week. My children and grandchildren all live out of town. A phone call to any one of my grandchildren always lifts my spirits. Their energy is contagious, even over the phone."—Kathy, Michigan

"I try to look for the humor in an otherwise difficult situation, to make myself and others laugh, and to remind us all to not take ourselves too seriously. Laughter is the best medicine and a unifying force in the midst of stress." —Sue P., RN

"I think my staff is just the greatest. When our work life becomes very challenging I like to have lunch with the staff and catch up on what is happening in their home lives. It does help maintain balance. We lunch and learn that life does not have to be all serious."—Mary Ann, RN, BSN, MHA, OCN, Pittsburgh, PA

Resources on therapeutic writing

These books focus on the potential of writing to help people work through stressful situations:

Opening Up: The Healing Power of Expressing Emotions, by James W. Pennebaker. Sarasota, FL: The Guilford Press, 1997.

Writing to Heal: A Guided Journal for Recovering from Trauma & Emotional Upheaval, by James W. Pennebaker. Oakland, CA: New Harbinger Publications, 2004.

The Writing Cure: How Expressive Writing Promotes Health and Emotional Well-Being, Edited by Stephen J. Lepore and Joshua M. Smyth. Washington, DC: American Psychological Association, 2002.

Thriving Through Crisis: Turn Tragedy and Trauma into Growth and Change, by Bill O'Hanlon. New York: Perigee Trade, 2005.

To learn more about the full *Nursing Journal* workbook, including how to get a copy, visit www.josieking.org or email nursing@josieking.org.